IGOR KLIBANOV

STOP EXERCISING!

THE WAY YOU ARE DOING IT NOW.

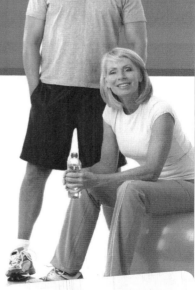

7 DANGEROUS FACTS

THAT WILL BACKFIRE AND CAUSE YOU TO STAY FAT OR HURT YOURSELF

D1070086

Author: Igor Klibanov
Title: STOP EXERCISING! The Way You Are Doing it Now
ISBN: 978-1-927411-52-0
Category: HEALTH & FITNESS / General

Publisher:
Black Card Books™
Division of Gerry Robert Enterprises Inc.
Suite 214
5-18 Ringwood Drive
Stouffville, Ontario
Canada, L4A 0N2
International Calling: 1-647-361-8577
www.blackcardbooks.com

- HUGH CONNOR
- PENNY / DU BARDOLO.

Table of Contents

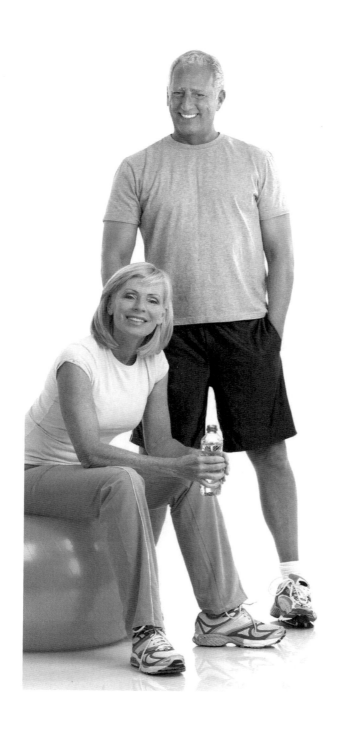

Foreword

By: Briana Santoro, CNP, NNCP, BBA (hons.)
Certified Nutritionist, No. 1 Best Selling Author of
Get Naked In The Kitchen, Owner of The Naked Label,
and Passionate Public Speaker

When I first met Igor I knew I had met a companion in natural health. His passion for helping people achieve their health goals radiates from. I was excited to learn about this book because the topics discussed in the following pages uncover very important information about how to achieve the health we really want.

I am a certified nutritionist and a lover of whole, natural foods, and dancing in the kitchen. Earlier in my career, I noticed that many clients who came to see me had an understanding of what they should do to reach their health goals but they weren't taking action. They would tell me what their goals were; then they would tell me what they ate that day, and I would ask them what was one thing they could have eaten different that would have been more aligned with their goals. They could always tell me at least one thing. It was then that I realized that information was important, but helping clients turn that information into action was essential for achieving the health they wanted. I found that truly transforming their relationship with food was what was needed and this has been a focus of mine ever since. One of the things I love about *STOP EXERCISING! The Way You Are Doing It Now* is that Igor has done a fantastic job of both providing information to show you what to do, as well as helping you uncover why you struggle to take action. I believe that it's this balance between information, motivation, and transformation that will be an important key to your success.

The other thing I love so much about this book is that it addresses the whole picture. So often, when people set a goal, they go out and take "some" actions. For example, if someone wants to lose weight the most common action is to eat less or to "go on a diet". The problem is that this is a short-term solution which doesn't fully address the underlying reason why you are overweight in the first place and it doesn't take into account all of the reasons why you gained the weight. This book takes a look at the whole picture. It looks at all the factors that are involved in reaching your health goals. It shows you not only how to reach your goals but, more important how to maintain that new fit and fabulous you!

Introduction

The alarm clock goes off before sunrise; you drag yourself out of bed and put on your running shoes, for your regular five-km run. You feel fantastic when you get home. You sit down to enjoy your healthy breakfast, and you are sure that when you get on the scale at the end of this week you will finally see the results you crave. Time and time again you swear that your scale *must* be broken — it can't be telling you that you have put on another pound. It has been a long time since you fell for that, *"Someone's got to eat the last doughnut,"* trick. After all, you didn't eat that last dipped doughnut which was sitting on the plate in the lunchroom last week. How is it possible to gain fat when you are exercising and eating right? What is going on?

You have picked just the right book to shed some light on your problem and you can be rest-assured that you are not alone. I wrote this book because most of our clients are busy, stressed-out professionals with children between the ages of 12-30 years old. Some of these clients are on some sort of medication. They exercise regularly and eat what they think is a healthy diet, but they are frustrated because they aren't seeing the fat-loss results they desire. The reason people come to us for help is because other fat-loss approaches have failed. We are only happy to help.

Fat loss is not just about exercise and nutrition. In my experience as a fitness professional, personal trainer, and public speaker I have discovered that *stress management* is critical to fat loss.

When most people think of exercise they think of long-duration cardiovascular exercise, such as swimming, running or cycling; although these activities may be enjoyable, they may also cause adrenal fatigue, which could be harming your fat-loss efforts. Then, we must consider the question of hormonal balance, digestive health, and the influence of toxins on the body. I have identified eight hidden reasons as to why some clients do not lose body fat despite doing everything right. I discuss this extensively on my website: 8hiddenreasons.com.

Body transformation is a combination of four factors: nutrition, supplementation, lifestyle, and exercise. In this book, I have drawn on the expertise of many other professionals in each field in order to give you the answers you seek.

The way my company works is that we assess our clients using our Symptom Questionnaire, Biosignature Modulation (which is a system of correlating your body fat to your hormonal profile) and, together with blood work, we find that they have one or more of the above-mentioned factors that point to fat-loss resistance. We will discuss fat loss as a pleasant side-effect of getting healthier, which may result in more energy: you will fit back into your clothes, and start noticing changes when you look in the mirror and, in turn, regain your self-confidence. Sound good?

Learn how to exercise, eat,
and supplement - for you.

Contact Fitness Solutions Plus!
www.torontofitnessonline.com

"Safe and effective fat loss involves an integrated approach that combines exercise, nutrition, supplements and lifestyle."

IGOR KLIBANOV
Author | Speaker | Fitness Professional

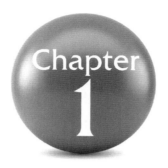

Is Stress Making Your Pants Tight?

You've tried blaming the dryer for your shrinking pants, but no one would believe you. It's time to face the truth: your pants are getting tighter and you have to find a legitimate reason for it. In the first chapter, we will discuss possible reasons for the mysterious shrinking of your pants and the prime suspect is: **stress**.

Igor Klibanov

Fat loss is about more than just calories. Hormones determine where you store body fat more than the amount of calories you ingest. On one side of the fat-loss scale (no pun intended) you have the Type 1 diabetes male or female who could consume over their daily requirement in calories, but would fade away without their insulin. On the other end of the scale, so to speak, is the person who has hypothyroidism or anemia and may only consume 1,000 calories a day, but they continue to store body fat. Why does this happen? Let's look at some factors that may contribute to this.

"You don't just need to lose weight to be healthy. You need to first be healthy to lose weight."
DIANA SCHWARZBEIN, M.D., from Santa Barbara, California

Dr. Diana Schwarzbein, who wrote *The Schwarzbein Principle*, is a graduate from the University of Southern California (USC) Medical School. She sub-specializes in metabolism, diabetes, osteoporosis, menopause, and thyroid conditions. Her idea that health precedes fat loss makes so much sense, and she is not alone in her view. Dr. Lise Janelle, an excellent psychotherapist from the *Centre For Heart Living* even goes so far as to say, "The more emphasis on weight-loss, the more stress it creates. The best thing is to focus on being healthy."

This goes in line with what Dr. John Berardi, PhD teaches. He is the co-founder and Chief Science Officer of *Precision Nutrition* and sits on the health and performance advisory boards of *Nike, Titleist, and Equinox*. Dr. Berardi's body transformation program, *Precision Nutrition* is one of the largest, most successful companies in the world. He says that you cannot control your weight; you can only control the habits that influence your weight. The idea behind this is that if you focus on being healthy, fat loss will come naturally as a side-effect. Look at it this way: even if you don't decrease your body-fat percentage, you can still improve your health without increasing your weight. It is a win-win situation. Perhaps a shift in focus is in order; good health should be the goal.

When we think of mental and emotional stress, we think of the guy down the street whose wife has left him or we recall the tension between family members at the annual family gathering. You may think the only stresses you experience are the ones your boss imposes on you; you may also be dealing with tight deadlines and other workplace anxieties.

What are the biggest reasons for fat-loss resistance? Michelle Armstrong, a nutritionist in Oakville, Ont., went so far as to say that stress management was one of the biggest reasons why some find it impossible to lose body fat. Clinical nutritionist, Dr. Robert Rakowski, who is also a chiropractor out of Houston Tex., and who gives seminars for Metagenics, concurs. Michelle Waithe, a holistic nutritionist from Nature's Emporium, who specifically works with diabetics, emphasizes how important stress management is to blood sugar regulation. We all agree that stress management is critical to solving the puzzle of resistance to fat loss.

Let's talk a little bit more about the origins of our stress responses. It is good to understand that our bodies can't tell the difference between mental or emotional stress and physical stress. Let us take a trip back in time to when humans were primarily hunters and gatherers— they lived off the land.

If we think back to the days when saber-tooth tigers roamed the earth, ready to make a meal out of one unsuspecting human wanderer, our bodies were primed to respond to such threats. You may have heard this response described as the "fight-or-flight" response. What would happen upon encountering the beast is your blood sugar would rise. This would happen because the body wants to have a fuel source ready for when you need to run away from the said tiger. Your blood pressure would rise temporarily, in order to pump blood to the muscles needed, while you would have made a quick escape from the threat. As long as you ran faster than the guy next to you, you had a fairly good chance of survival; it was about survival-of-the-fittest after all.

In contrast, nowadays, when we experience a deadline or some other stressful event, we experience the same physical response as if we were back in those days. The physical response is there, but your body does not follow-up with the running and fighting scenario, because if you treated your boss that way, you'd be fired! Although we have the same physiological response, the blood sugar has nowhere to go, so blood sugar stays high as a result of not being used as fuel, as it might have been in the prehistoric era.

You may have heard about a well-known primatologist, Robert M. Sapolsky, and author of the book, *Why Zebras Don't Get Ulcers.* He pointed out that most of us do not lie awake at night worrying about whether we have some tropical disease like malaria or the bubonic plague. Instead, the diseases we fear are silent killers such as heart disease and cancer. When we worry or experience stress, our body turns on the same physiological responses as an animal's does; we no longer need, however, to react to stress in the same way as an animal would, through fighting or fleeing so that over time our stress response literally makes us sick.

Let's look at the mechanics of what happens in the body when we're under stress. Blood pressure rises; we start to perspire and Cortisol, which is a hormone, is released into the bloodstream. Every hormone in your body affects other hormones; they are in a complicated, continual state of flux as one or more hormones is released; they affect one another and, in turn, regulate the workings of the body. The release of Cortisol affects other hormones, such as those released by the thyroid, plus other key hormones such as testosterone, estrogen, insulin, and leptin.

Can stress really have such a bad effect on me? Isn't *everyone* under stress nowadays? We'll discuss this in more detail in a few moments, but first let's look at the symptoms that may present themselves when you are under stress. If your doctor is on your case about your high blood sugar or high blood pressure, which are common side-effects of stress, you may want to sit up and pay attention. What is your body telling you? You may encounter feelings of hopelessness and fatigue.

People who are under stress often find themselves unable to get a good night's sleep. Stress may take on one of two forms of appetite adjustment - either there is a significant loss of appetite or an increase in appetite - both of those responses are symptoms of stress. Feeling light-headed when going from lying to sitting, or sitting to standing is an indicator that something is up, in case you didn't notice the prominent dark circles under your eyes every morning. All is not lost. Now that we know what stress looks like, it is good to know that the degree to which stress is damaging to your system depends on how you handle it.

Everyone is under some degree of stress. It is easy to place financial concern under the category of stress-related factors, but there are some elements that influence our stress levels with which we may not be aware. Those include: poor nutrition, too much or too little exercise, radiation, pollution, and environmental influences.

Now you have proof that all this stress is the culprit for your tight pants. Since you might be pulling out your hair in frustration anyway, let's send off a sample of hair to Dr. Jennifer Cisternino for analysis. Diagnostic testing helps to find out exactly which hormones and minerals are out of balance or depleted due to the effects of stress, and a hair mineral analysis is a good way to go. I know you're wondering what happens if you're bald. Well, you will be pleased to know there are ways to get around that. The hair sample is analyzed for different nutrients after you provide the appropriate information about the type of shampoo you use. Time to confess if you colour your hair and, also, you will be asked whether you swim in chlorine swimming pools or not.

The analysis will provide information about the levels of toxic minerals such as mercury, lead, calcium, magnesium, chromium and other minerals. They look at the ratios between different nutrients. Also, shining a light into the eyes from the side and noting the response of the pupil - the pupillary response - is an indicator of adrenal dysfunction, unless you have been dabbling in illegal drugs, which will also affect your adrenals, so they do go hand-in-hand.

In addition to hair mineral analysis, Dr. Jennifer Cisternino uses other low-tech tests. One of those is orthostatic hypotension. In this test, your blood pressure is measured after five minutes of lying down and relaxing, and then blood pressure is once again measured immediately after standing up. Typically, it should rise 6-10 mmHg; if it drops or stays the same it is in indicator that there may be problems with the adrenal glands.

Dr. Andrea Maxim likes to use the Metagenics Identi-T stress profile. This is a profile used to categorize different stress responses; in other words, different people react to stress in different ways. The Identi-T Stress profiles:

- *Stressed and wired*
- *Stressed and tired*
- *Stressed and hot*
- *Stressed and cold*

- *Stressed and immune challenged (you catch colds when under stress)*

- *Stressed and mentally exhausted (either a racing mind, or inability to think)*

All the ladies ask me where the chocolate response fits in. That is another subject altogether. Victoria Lorient-Fabish, a holistic psychotherapist, speaker, and life-and-wellness coach said that anxiety can be a problematic mental block because it will cause people to seek out comfort foods. So there you go!

Dr. Andrea Maxim also uses urine testing as a diagnostic tool and then she matches up the appropriate herb or adaptogen which fits your particular stress profile so that the treatment is precise. The urine test is used to determine the client's levels of sodium, potassium, and chloride.

First, you need to rebalance your body chemistry before fat loss is a possibility. If your symptoms and/or blood work point to the fact that your biochemistry is out of balance, then you may not respond to weight loss. I have seen this time and time again as a fitness professional.

Yes, you may be resistant to fat loss, even if you're eating right and exercising. First, you need to rebalance your body chemistry before fat loss is a possibility.

Josh Gitalis, a clinical nutritionist and instructor at the *Institute of Holistic Nutrition*, says that he doesn't treat fat loss directly. He maintains that fat is a symptom of other things going on in the body. He says that once health-related issues are dealt with, fat loss is a side-effect. I wholeheartedly agree because I see it with many of my clients.

The stressed-out individual, who has been diagnosed by using both a combination of symptom analysis and blood work, needs to participate in a certain kind of exercise to see results. These light activities include tai chi and walking. What would *not* be ideal would be long-duration cardiovascular exercise; high-intensity cardio is not advisable for somebody who has this profile.

This reiterates my point that hormones determine fat loss more than calories because, although long-duration cardio will burn more calories than a low-intensity exercise, such as jogging versus walking, lighter activities will speed up fat-burning in the client with this kind of profile.

If you have been diagnosed with adrenal fatigue you should eat minimally-processed carbohydrates. We say "*no*" to white bread, but "*yes*" to potatoes because of elevated cortisol levels in this case. Carbohydrates stimulate insulin. Dr. Dianna Schwarzbein pointed out that insulin is a fat-storing hormone. Therefore, it makes perfect sense that if your insulin is out of balance, you will store fat more easily.

Cortisol and insulin are antagonistic hormones. One lowers blood sugar, while the other one elevates it. Eating moderate carbohydrates will bring blood sugar down. When insulin rises, cortisol falls like a teeter-totter. Cortisol raises blood sugar. Insulin lowers blood sugar.

Eat your moderate carbohydrates when your cortisol is high and I suggest you figure out when that is by getting a salivary cortisol test done.Cortisol has natural highs and lows throughout the day. That's called your "cortisol rhythm." Healthy cortisol rhythm is high cortisol in the morning and low in the evening. If you have adrenal fatigue you do not have a healthy cortisol rhythm. You may have different rhythms; in some cases, you may have a reverse rhythm, where you are tired in the morning, with a second-wind at night, or you may encounter some other sort of fluctuation.

The times of day when you feel most energetic are likely when you have the highest cortisol levels. I like to use the combination of symptom analysis, Biosignature, and laboratory testing.

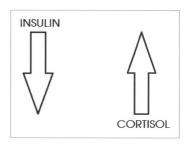

What are the correct supplements to take when you are stressed? Dr. Makoto Trotter said that if the stress you're feeling won't go away (you're not going to quit your job), use adaptogens to help – these are specific herbs that can increase your cortisol when it is low, or decrease it when it is high.

Both Dr. Tara Andresen and Dr. Andrea Maxim put their clients on a combination of the B-complex, vitamin B5 (on top of what's found in the B-complex) and vitamin C.

These are three of the five nutrients that are depleted the most when people are under stress; another supplement to consider taking is magnesium in fairly high dosages. This course of action is not forever – just until adrenal fatigue is remedied. Hang on a moment – before you go out scouring the health-store shelves for these supplements, let me just warn you: self-diagnosis or self-medicating is not advised and I strongly suggest you consult a professional in this area.

Adaptogens are herbs that help you adapt to stress.

Examples:

- *Ashwagandha*

- *Holy basil*

- *Ginseng*

- *Rhodiola*

- *Licorice*

- *Cordyceps*

How do you figure out what's a high-quality supplement and what's not? It's beyond the scope of this book, but I've previously written about it on my blog. Check it out at this link:

www.fitnesssolutionsplus.ca/nutritional-supplement/

Sleep is a vital and important part of the recovery process and we advise clients to get at least10 hours of sleep a day during the recovery phase, particularly from 11 p.m. to 9 a.m. I asked Dr. Spencer Nadolsky, an osteopathic doctor, what is the first thing he looks at when a client comes to him wanting fat loss and his answer was, "Sleep." He starts his clients off with questions on sleep.

He wants to know how many hours of sleep you get. Is it good sleep? Is there snoring? Do you suffer from sleep apnea? Do you feel tired? He inquires about the quality of sleep, whether the client feels tired when they wake up or well-rested, and so on. "We always check for sleep apnea, because if a client has it, they won't be able to lose weight easily even if they are eating right and exercising," says Dr. Nadolsky.

Igor Klibanov

Dr. John Dempster says, "If you're not sleeping, you're not resetting or repairing your endocrine system." Melatonin is one of the key hormones that regulate sleep, but it also affects other hormones in the body.

Hans Selye, in the book, *"The Stress of Life,"* talks about perception having more effect on the body than reality. People, for example, who are afraid of flying. If they feel the slightest bit of turbulence, they take narcotics to calm themselves down. A child, on the other hand, feels the same turbulence and likens it to a fun roller-coaster ride. We see a good example of a different perception during the same event.

We can use the same analogy when comparing someone with arachnophobia (fear of spiders) and someone who does not care what a spider on the wall is doing or where it is headed. Two onlookers with different threat perceptions, will react physically in two very different ways. Hans encourages people to work on perception. What's stressful to one person may not be stressful to another; therefore, it is important to note that perception matters. Look for the positive in different situations. When under stress, make a plan to solve problems. Write your plan down. This helps you see the light at the end of the tunnel.

Another good stress management technique is to make a plan to solve the problem of stress because stress can be seen as an abstract problem until you identify it and address it head on. Give it a name! Sometimes it is not the circumstances that are causing you stress, but their abstract nature, or your lack of clarity, or control over it. Make a plan to solve it; write down that plan, which helps you to see the proverbial light at the end of the tunnel. It helps to give stress a form and a shape so that you can deal with it and plan to solve the problem or, at least, cope better.

Take This Quick Self-Evaluation Test

Here is a simple self-evaluation test you can use to estimate the degree to which you are affected by all of these factors.

 What is my perceived level of stress? Rate yourself on a scale of 0 to 10. (0 being 'no perceived stress,' 10 'feeling overwhelmed and ready to pull your hair out.')

Make a mark on the line where you think you fit in.

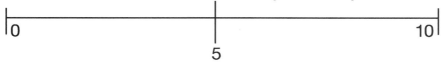

Igor Klibanov

 How am I sleeping? Do I have a regular, healthy sleep pattern? Do I fall asleep right away or does it take me a long time to fall asleep? When I wake up do I feel refreshed or tired and could sleep another couple of hours? Are there any lights in my bedroom? Do I need to get up to use the washroom at night? (0 is good sleep; 10 indicated no sleep at all.)

Make a mark on the line where you think you fit in.

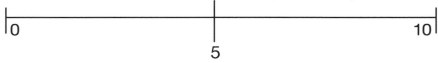

Note: *Moonlight, alarm clock digits, and any other light should be blocked out as much as possible. Electronic devices should, ideally, not be in the bedroom. Yes, I am talking about the smartphone on your side table and your laptop. These should all be outside the bedroom. No televisions or cellphones (even if they are turned off) in the bedroom so that you can optimize your sleep experience. Here's an example: I asked a client who was always on the go and always went to work at 5 a.m. to sleep in. Two weeks later his calves were leaner, but what was even more impressive was that he lost six mm, in two weeks, of belly fat when measured with my calipers. He had made no other changes.*

Evaluate Your Nutrition

 Am I eating seven servings of fruit and vegetables a day? (½ cup is one serving) (10 indicates that you eat all servings in a typical day; 0 will indicate none eaten.)

Make a mark on the line where you think you fit in.

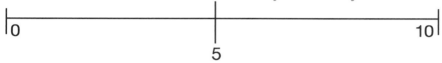

 Am I eating at least three servings (a serving is about the size of the palm of your hand) of meat, fish, or seafood a day? (10 indicates required consumption; 0 indicates vegetarianism or vegan lifestyle.)

Make a mark on the line where you think you fit in.

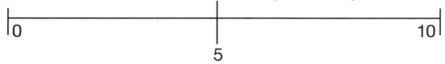

Why those three? Meat, fish, or seafood are the best sources of lean protein. Some may argue that cheese or eggs, or beans are proteins but I don't consider those to be primary sources of protein. Yes, beans do have protein in them. A cup of beans may have 16-18 grams of protein in them; however, they also have 38-40 grams of carbohydrates per cup. It is not that it is bad - it certainly is healthy for you - but I don't consider beans to be a source of protein. Eggs are a great source of protein, but an ever better source of saturated fat.

27

That is just the way it is; I recommend eggs but I would not consider them a source of lean protein. Is this restrictive? My answer is "No," because just within the meat category you have chicken, turkey, beef, veal, pork, lamb, and more. Then you have a wide variety of fish and seafood that you can have.

 Am I ingesting any stimulants such as caffeine and alcohol or sweeteners and sugar? (10 indicates you don't use coffee, alcohol and sugar; 0 indicates that you can't live without them.)

Make a mark on the line where you think you fit in.

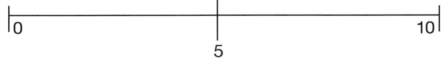

0   5   10

We will discuss food sensitivities in more detail in Chapter 2, but do you have any food sensitivities? Food sensitivities will affect stress management. Example: Biosignature Modulation profiles indicate your hormonal profile by looking at where you store fat. Based on this, a client of mine cut out coffee and made no other changes. Her fat measurement dropped around her belly just by cutting out that particular stimulant. When this same client increased protein, she lost fat over her triceps but nowhere else. By the way, your knee measurement goes down when you cut out alcohol.

Q *Am I participating in high-intensity activities or moderate-intensity activities for long durations of time? (Cardio, like swimming, cycling, jogging etcetera. 0 means not at all, and 10 means six days a week or more).*

Make a mark on the line where you think you fit in.

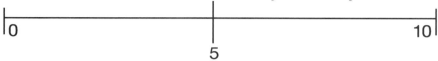

Although exercise can alleviate stress mentally by the release of endorphins and so on, if you are over-training you are placing a certain amount of stress on the body. Many find long-duration activities are very enjoyable, but the physiological effect it can have on the body can cause the same response as the "fight-or-flight" reaction. I don't advise giving up your favourite activity, but I do recommend that activities which may be causing adrenal fatigue be put on hold until you are well on your way to recovery. I never advise long-duration cardio for fat loss; however, some people just enjoy it for its own sake, in which case I don't tell them to stop.

Q *Am I taking High quality Supplements? (10 indicates high quality supplements from a health store, 0 indicates none taken, not ever.)*

Make a mark on the line where you think you fit in.

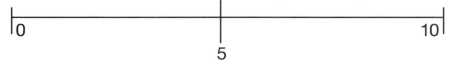

Igor Klibanov

If you want to know more about how to determine supplement quality, see this link:

www.fitnesssolutionsplus.ca/nutritional-supplement/

 Could I improve my time-management skills? (0 indicates well-organized lifestyle with minimal stress: you are always on time. 10 indicates that you are always flying by the seat of your pants and life is one continual emotional roller-coaster of deadlines and stress; you are always late for appointments.)

Make a mark on the line where you think you fit in.

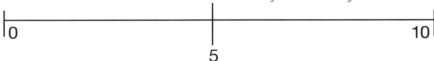

0   5   10

Time-management issues can be resolved; it is a matter of choice. For example, one of my clients was a stressed-out marketing consultant. He was skinny, but had a high percentage of body fat. A year later his belly fat measurement had halved and I asked him what he had done differently as we weren't working together at that time. Without changing his nutrition or exercise, the one thing that he did change was how he was managing his schedule. His time management had improved, he was going to sleep earlier and waking up later, and his sleep was more restful. He lost 16 mm of belly fat in a year! (As measured with calipers.) Wow! That was not a fast fat loss but, considering he made no other changes, it is pretty impressive.

Many clients come back from a vacation thinking they must have gained body fat when, in fact, they don't or they have lost some due to the effect of relaxation and rest. This is also because they claim they aren't exercising, but they forget that playing tennis, golfing, scuba diving, walking, and hiking are all still exercises, even if you're not inside a gym setting.

Another client with a severe rotator cuff injury would not take supplements to help recover from injury; instead he went to Florida for six months and came back with the injury gone. His intake of natural vitamin C and vitamin D at his sunshine destination did the trick without him realizing it.

Q *Has my blood work been screened for possible deficiencies and imbalances in my blood chemistry? (10 indicates that you have had extensive diagnostic blood work, 0 indicating you have never had diagnostic blood work.)*

Make a mark on the line where you think you fit in.

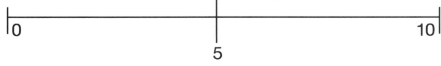

0

5

10

In introducing blood work screening to my clients, I have seen that we often pick up on important indicators that doctors missed. We look at the difference between optimal and "normal."

Problems with modern blood chemistry occur because each lab may have different standards where reference ranges and markers are not standardized.

Labs use the blood work of those who come in for blood work to determine their reference ranges; they use the blood work results of those who are coming in because they are sick or unhealthy. As a result, they are good at catching disease, but not so good at measuring health. Lack of adequate markers is also a problem, since fewer markers are being covered by health insurance. Now that you know about these important factors you know what may be contributing to the mysterious shrinkage of your pants. See where these principles may apply to you. It is a lot to take in and should you need the help of a professional, take advantage of the free Dream Body MAP session at the end of the book (which has a value of $319.00).

If you don't want to be that stressed-out person who looks older than they actually are, write out your list of follow-up steps. If most of your self-evaluation answers were between 0-5 on the scale, there is room for improvement. Based on your self-evaluation take the steps necessary to improve your sleep, deal with stress, and focus on getting healthier. When these principles are applied under the supervision of a professional, together, we can expect that your pants will become loose again and you may even get to go shopping for a smaller pair.

Learn how to exercise, eat, and supplement - for you.

Contact Fitness Solutions Plus!

www.torontofitnessonline.com

"Lose 10, 20, 50 pounds or more without starving yourself, counting calories or using willpower. And do it all safely, without getting hurt in the process."

IGOR KLIBANOV
Author | Speaker | Fitness Professional

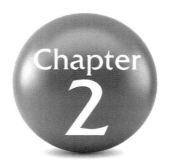

Chapter

2

Is Weight Gain Giving You a Belly Ache?

T he subject of digestive health is a fun one, isn't it? Be warned, there is no easy way to talk about digestion without getting into a little bit of TMI (Too Much Information), but I will do my best to keep it as polite as possible. After all, it is strictly on a 'need-to-know' basis, and *you need to know.* We all eat food that has to be digested, so here we go!

Igor Klibanov

Why does poor digestive health affect weight loss?

When we talk about digestive health, we will focus on the stomach, small intestine, and large intestine. The liver, although not part of the gastrointestinal system, needs to be included in this discussion because the liver plays an important role in the detoxification of the body. Each one of these organs has a distinct role to play in the process of digestion which in turn affects fat loss. As Clinical Nutritionist, Josh Gitalis says, "Digestion is where everything begins and ends." Digestion starts in the mouth when we take our first bite and start to chew.

"Digestion is where everything begins and ends."
JOSH GITALIS

Stomach

When food is swallowed, the journey of digestion begins and saliva helps to carry food to the stomach. When your food moves into the stomach, it then encounters hydrochloric acid; this very strong acid prepares your food for the process where nutrients are then absorbed in the intestines. Hydrochloric acid breaks down protein. Protein is broken down into amino acids, which are the building blocks of the protein molecule. That means that amino acids are responsible for strength and repair inside the body. Hydrochloric acid enables nutrients such as zinc, B12, calcium, magnesium and iron to be extracted from your food. If the stomach has an *insufficient* amount of this stomach acid, this process is impeded and, instead, your lunch putrefies. This does not sound so good does it? When these important nutrients are not extracted properly and sufficiently, health problems may occur.

Vitamin B12 is needed for energy production. It is a water-soluble vitamin needed for the synthesis and regulation of fatty acids. We need calcium and magnesium for our dental and skeletal health as well as for proper nerve conduction. We need B12 to keep our brain and nervous system healthy. When these essential nutrients are not extracted and absorbed by the body, due to insufficient stomach acid, problems begin to occur.

Canadian, Charles Poliquin, who has trained numerous Olympic athletes is an internationally-renowned strength coach. He invented BioSignature Modulation, a reliable method of highly specific and science-based approach to hormone assessment, which I use for the benefit of my clients. It was from Charles Poliquin that I learned the principle that the closer to the mouth problems occur in the digestive system, the more the effects will be felt further south in the digestive processes.

Igor Klibanov

Small Intestine

The small intestine aids in the extraction of remaining nutrients from the food you ingested. Absorption takes place through the walls of the small intestine. In this part of the intestine we encounter both friendly and unfriendly bacteria.

Clinical nutritionist, Dr. Robert Rakowski, said something about bacteria that I have paraphrased here: 'that good bugs eat food and eliminate (read "poop") nutrients'; Bad bugs eat nutrients and eliminate (yup, read "poop" again) toxins. Frank Roberts said, "A lot of times, it's not an issue of toxicity, but deficiency, because deficiencies will allow toxins to infiltrate."

Here's a little bit of interesting information: 80 to 90 percent of the body's serotonin, a neurotransmitter which helps prevent depression by regulating your mood, is found in the small intestine; because of this it has been nicknamed our "second brain." Our immune system is aimed at the small intestine to seek and destroy foreign invaders.

Just imagine all those bad bacteria in a little war inside your small intestine—sounds a lot like an epic video game. If your intestinal bacteria balance is off, then you can potentially be too toxic—in other words, the "bad guys" are winning.

How you feel influences how you eat, and how you eat influences how you feel. Practitioners will often treat patients with depression by first treating their digestive system before moving on to further treatment.

Large Intestine

The large intestine or colon is where water is separated from undigested food. It is also the last step before elimination. Sodium and potassium are antagonistic minerals, so their proportions to each other will regulate how much water is retained or excreted. If you have a slow metabolism or hypothyroidism, elimination is delayed. Just as you have transit time when you are travelling on vacation, your food has a transit time as it passes through your digestive system. In other words, the time it takes to travel from mouth to anus. Your food's 'travel time' should be from 18 to 24 hours.

There is a very simple test you can perform to find out whether your food takes the concord or the slow train to its final destination. Examine the resulting gastric output when you eat beets or corn. Make a note of how long it takes to pass. This will indicate your own personal digestive transit time. Friendly bacteria play an important role in transit time as Jason Tetro, author of *The Germ Code* explains: "If excreting sooner than 12 hours, or longer than 24 hours, it means you have a deficiency." If food stays in the digestive tract too long it putrefies and releases toxins; natural toxins, but they are toxins nonetheless. This delay in peristalsis, which is a series of wave-like muscle contractions that moves food to different processing stations in the digestive tract, can slow down fat loss. Let's go back to your Grade 7 biology class for a moment. Mitochondria are parts of a cell and their main function is to convert energy; they are often called the 'powerhouse' of the cell. Dr. Robert Rakowski pointed out that all toxins inhibit mitochondrial function. As a result, if the fat is not being burned off as energy, you will not be able to lose fat even if you are eating right and exercising.

The Liver

The liver is essentially the body's detoxification plant. This organ receives the most amount of blood flow at rest. If the body thinks that the liver is *that* important, it must place a high priority on the detoxification process. The liver balances blood sugar, as well as manages toxins and hormones. The liver produces bile, while the gall bladder stores and releases it. Bile helps the body to emulsify fat. The liver has important functions in the healthy working of the body and that is why it is so important to look after your liver. Be kind to this little organ - don't overdo the wild parties. If your liver is not functioning properly, you will not lose body fat—even if you are exercising and eating well. We use a combination of blood work and hair mineral analysis with our clients to screen for potential liver problems. To learn how to assess the liver function is beyond the scope of the book, but you can see us for your own Dream Body MAP Session. (See page 125-126)

How do you know if your digestive health is poor?

If your digestive health is not as it should be you may experience some of the following symptoms: heartburn, burping, or gas an hour after eating, plus diarrhea or bad breath.

Another symptom is the occurrence of foul smelling sweat due to the body attempting to rid itself of toxins through the skin, which is one of the body's largest detoxification organs. You may experience bloating one to two hours after eating. If your stomach is upset by greasy foods, this may also indicate potential digestive problems.

The last symptom we will discuss is constipation, which is considered to be less than one bowel movement a day, or if you have two or three but they are difficult or painful to pass. Here is where the TMI comes in; a normal, healthy stool should be toothpaste consistency without a strong odour. Since we are being frank about this, a healthy person should pass about a foot of excrement a day. I know, an awkward subject, but you've got to know. If you don't know, you will not know what to look for. Subject closed!

In order to gauge whether you have sufficient stomach acid you can do the Betaine HCl challenge test – this involves a controlled regimen of this supplement that helps maintain stomach acid, taken orally during a meal. We thoroughly assess our clients with a 321-symptom questionnaire to find out if they have poor digestive health. Take advantage of our Dream Body MAP session offer at the back of the book. (See page 125-126).

The 4R program, which helps to restore digestive health, was formulated by Jeffrey Bland, PhD, biochemist, and father of Functional Medicine.

Remove:
- *Toxins (eat organic)*
- *Sensitivities (get tested with IgG, or go for the most common ones: gluten, dairy, sugar, corn).*

Replace:
- *Betaine HCl*
- *Enzymes*

Reinoculate:
- *Probiotics and prebiotics*

Repair:
- *Glutamine*

Remove

Dr. Makoto Trotter, ND, suggested that you figure out what food sensitivities are keeping the inflammation cycle in your gut since that is yet another stress on the body.

The difference between a food allergy and sensitivity is simply this: if you have an allergy, the reaction is severe and immediate. If you have food sensitivity the reaction is subtle and delayed. Our goal is to eliminate both from your diet. Although people tend to automatically eliminate foods to which they are allergic because of the symptoms that occur, rarely do we pay attention to food sensitivities. This is because the effects of the foods ingested are subtle and we often do not make the connection with the delayed symptoms. Some of these symptoms include nasal congestion a few hours after eating or achy body the following day.

In order to investigate food sensitivities in my clients, I prefer to use the IgG test which is a laboratory test that will accurately pinpoint food sensitivities. The IgG test lists approximately 200 different foods.

If you prefer to not do the lab test, then you can go the route of doing an elimination diet. The downside of this option, although it may cost a lot less, is that you

Igor Klibanov

have to exercise self-discipline. To accurately find out what you are sensitive to, you *have* to eliminate the most common allergens for the two-week test period. This means reading labels and being very careful about what you eat. That leaves you with plenty of vegetables (except for potatoes, tomatoes, bell peppers, egg plants, corn, and chili peppers), most meats (except pork), and most nuts and seeds, in addition to all fruit. You can eat any of these in unlimited quantities. You should not go hungry—this is important.

If you have no time or patience for either option, eliminate the most common allergens in North America which are gluten, dairy, sugar, corn, and soy. This is the least-preferred option out of the three because it is not specific to your body or its needs.

Replace

Replace that which was lost, such as digestive enzymes and restore stomach acid. Be sure to take high-quality digestive enzymes which help with the digestion of proteins, carbohydrates, and fats. These are enzymes are protease, amylase, and lipase.

Reinoculate

Probiotics are friendly microorganisms that populate the small intestine, as we already discussed. You want to have more probiotics in your gut than bad bacteria.

Most companies do not produce high-quality probiotics. Choose a capsule that has between 15 and 60-billion live bacteria in it.

Many think of yogurt as a good source of probiotics, but it contains an inadequate number to make much difference to your intestinal population. Choose a product that is guaranteed at the time of expiry, *not* at the date of manufacture and packaging, because some bacteria die off before you consume the capsules. Different strains of bacteria have different lifespans.

Companies who make high-quality probiotics compensate for the anticipated loss of bacteria in the time it takes the product to get to consumers. Additional bacteria are placed into the product to ensure a high number of bacteria survive to do their job in your intestines. Check the product label for these very important words: "live and active cultures."

Prebiotics are the foods that probiotics eat! Feed those little guys what they need to survive and thrive. Prebiotics are found in bananas, honey, garlic, onions, and whole grains. If a person is working on killing some bad bacteria and Candida, it's important to avoid fruits for a period of time (one to three weeks). So get your prebiotics through supplements initially. Then you can switch to food sources.

Repair

It is essential that the lining of your digestive system is healthy. If there has been any damage, healing and repair need to take place before proper digestion and health can be maintained. The stomach has a coating around it which prevents it from being worn-out by the highly acidic hydrochloric acid, which can burn through a car hood if poured onto a car. Glutamine helps to repair stomach lining. In addition to glutamine you can use DGL (*Deglycerrized* licorice) and aloe vera to repair the digestive lining. Nutritionist, Michelle Armstrong said, "You're going to have a very hard time losing fat if you're chronically inflamed. If one thing's off, it throws everything off."

In conclusion, it is essential to improve and maintain your digestive health. In taking steps to do so, you will reap the benefits and your body will thank you for it.

The 4R's

Remove	Replace	Reinoculate	Repair

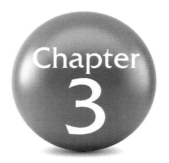

Chapter 3

Hormones More Important than Calories

This chapter will not include snide remarks about women and their roller-coaster hormones, so it is safe to proceed. I do, however, want to stress that hormones are responsible for the storage of body fat, more so than calories. First order of business is to balance your hormones, and fat loss will be a pleasant side-effect. There is a hormonal hierarchy, in terms of how much control you have over them and insulin is first on the list. The second most controllable hormone is cortisol and we are thankful for that little hormone when we are able to react in a crisis as discussed in chapter one.

Insulin and cortisol are the two primary hormones which need to be controlled as a prerequisite for all other hormones to function properly. It doesn't matter if you have imbalances in estrogen, thyroid, testosterone, and so on; if these first two are out of balance, the other hormones will not be restored. If insulin and cortisol are working as they should and there are still imbalances in testosterone, estrogen, thyroid, and so on then by all means go after them directly.

Hormonal Imbalance

To determine imbalances in insulin and cortisol in our clients, we use a combination of symptom identification and blood work. The reason we combine these two approaches in tandem is because everyone is different and some people do not present symptoms at all. One client who filled out our extensive questionnaire was asymptomatic; in other words, he presented no symptoms of high insulin. Based on his BioSignature profile, his waist circumference indicated otherwise. Upon doing his blood work, we found he was diabetic without knowing it.

Insulin Imbalance

Symptoms for insulin imbalance include sugar cravings, irritability if meals are missed, frequent urination, or thirst. Sometimes clients experience shakiness if meals are missed. When clients have an insulin imbalance, often upon taking measurements we find that most fat is stored around the stomach and love-handle areas.

There are a few ways we can test for insulin levels and one of them is blood work. Routine blood test scores, however, are not good enough. (As discussed in Chapter 1) More extensive testing is necessary. Test for fasting glucose, fasting insulin, and HbA1C. The HbA1C test gives us an indication of how many hemoglobin cells have a sugar molecule bound to it. This test gives an idea of what your blood sugar is like over three to four months rather than the fasting glucose test, which is like a snapshot of what your blood sugar is like at the moment of drawing the blood sample. Glucose can be higher one hour earlier or one hour later than when you had the test done and therefore inaccurate.

Cortisol Imbalance

Symptoms for cortisol imbalance include lightheadedness when going from lying to standing, or low blood pressure. If you often crave a bag of salty chips or snacks, you might have cortisol imbalance. Further symptoms are dark circles under the eyes or constant fatigue. If you are a night owl you might want to have your cortisol levels checked. Another symptom of cortisol imbalance is that you store fat around the stomach and love handles.

There are some salivary tests for adrenal fatigue, but you can get an accurate reading with standard blood work. Testing for cortisol, DHEA-S, sodium, potassium, chloride, testosterone, and estrogen can help catch early-warning signs to prevent more serious problems down the line.

Balance Your Insulin

A simple way to balance your insulin is to ensure you get at least seven servings of vegetables a day. Each serving is a half cup or a handful. Get at least three servings of meat, fish, or seafood a day. Include 30 grams of fibre a day in addition to the vegetables. Choose from this list: flax seeds, chia seeds, hemp seeds, psyllium, and pectin. It is best to cycle these rather than using one for an extended period. I have seen good results with my clients who have done so; I have seen a marked drop in belly fat, love handle fat, and upper back fat - as much as 6-8 mm in caliper measurements. This result is significant since we take measurements bi-weekly.

Strength Training Is Paramount

The exercise regimen I follow with my clients for best results is a combination of strength and endurance training. Strength training is paramount in addressing insulin imbalance. Increased muscle mass can make you more sensitive to insulin and can lower blood sugar without the use of insulin; this is what is known as non-insulin mediated glucose transport.

If you are emaciated (extremely thin), then participate in less endurance training and include more strength training in your workout. If you are overweight, then combine an equal amount of endurance and strength training.

Suggested supplements you should take to help regulate insulin are chromium, magnesium glycinate, and B vitamins. I have been using medical foods instead of isolated nutrients and have been seeing good results. Medical foods are powders similar to protein powders, but without the same proteins. Medical foods have high doses of nutrients relative to a specific condition. There is a medical food for estrogen imbalance; there is another for blood sugar balance and so on. Each one has a different nutrient profile. One of the most popular topics at my speaking engagements is supplements and I am able to talk about this subject in great detail.

There are four criteria supplements must have in order to be called medical foods, which are:

- *Guaranteed potency (in other words, what they say is in the product is on the label)*

- *Guaranteed purity (no toxins, no traces of metals)*

- *Proven effectiveness in human clinical trials*

- *Every nutrient is regarded as safe; there is no fear of overdosing on any one nutrient.*

These products are government regulated and can only be obtained through health practitioners. Most local health store will not stock them.

Pavel Tsatsouline, former Soviet Special Forces physical training instructor, brought kettlebell training to North America in the late-1990s. He was in Russia and saw some men digging ditches with shovels and he asked the man in charge why they didn't just use a front-end loader. The answer was that they were creating jobs. Pavel's reply was, "Then why don't you give them spoons?" This illustration is a good explanation for why I like to use medical foods (the front end-loader of nutrition) rather than single, isolated nutrient supplements (spoons).

Balance Your Cortisol

As discussed in Chapter 1, stress management plays an important role in cortisol management. The hours of sleep between 11 p.m. and 9 a.m. are considered a very nourishing time for the body. For cortisol regulation, partake in very light exercise, like walking, stretching, tai chi, yoga, and so on because intense exercise stimulates cortisol production and taxes the adrenal glands. Heavy exercise is not recommended. If your cortisol levels are fine, you can't use this excuse and say, "Igor said so." Nice try!

Again, identify food sensitivities and remove them. Food sensitivities can affect your adrenal glands because when you eat foods to which you have a sensitivity, your body releases cortisol. There's a catch: these foods are sometimes the very same ones you crave! Most people have sensitivities to foods that they eat most frequently. Your brain releases very powerful chemicals or opioids, which are stronger than morphine, and which cause you to become addicted to these foods.

Upon eating said foods, your body releases a small amount of adrenalin (which feels good) and can result in addictive behaviour. It is important to eliminate these foods so that the adrenal glands can recover.

As I mentioned earlier, eat your starches at times of high cortisol. Supplement with a combination of B-complex, B5 and C. Use anti-inflammatory herbs and spices liberally, such as turmeric, cinnamon, ginger, and boswellia. Supplement your diet with herbs specific to *your* stress profile.

Why Do Menopausal Women Have A Hard Time?

Debra Waterhouse, author of *Outsmarting the Midlife Fat Cell*, maintains that women who do gain 4-10 lbs. during menopause, assuming they were not overweight to begin with, have better sleep and fewer symptoms associated with menopause. The three things that produce estrogen are the ovaries, body fat (the technical term is, adipocytes, or adipose tissue), and adrenal glands.

Now is your chance; you have the perfect excuse to add adrenal support in abundance during this time of life. Go to the spa, get a manicure, a massage, and go on vacation. Your body and your spouse will thank you for it.

What causes the most common problems in midlife is, first and foremost, an imbalance of cortisol and insulin and only secondarily imbalances in estrogen, progesterone, testosterone, etcetera. Balance your insulin and cortisol, and often the others take care of themselves.

When Testosterone and Estrogen Imbalances Remain After Fixing Adrenals and Insulin Levels

Supplement with B-complex vitamins. Zinc helps with testosterone balance, which both men and women need. Include plenty of cruciferous vegetables in your diet; these include cauliflower, cabbage, broccoli, bok choy, kale, cabbage, and collard greens.

Include coconut oil in your diet. It is a misconception that coconut oil is unhealthy. It is a healthy source of saturated fat which your body needs to make hormones.

When these hormones are already out of balance you need to give them a little extra support by supplying them with the building blocks or raw materials which are needed. Just to be clear, if you have high cholesterol to begin with; coconut oil is not a good choice for you.

Do an estrogen detoxification using:

- *DIM*

- *CDG*

- *Grapeseed extact*

- *Resveratrol*

DIM stands for diindolylmethane. It is a super antioxidant. CDG stands for Calcium-D-Glucarate. It's not calcium, as many people think. The liver has six detoxification pathways, and one of them is called "glucoronidation." This pathway, among other things, helps with estrogen detoxification. CDG stimulawtes this pathway. Grapeseed extract and resveratrol are phytonutrients (plant nutrients) and antioxidants that have a balancing effect on estrogen. In addition to these methods, I like to use medical foods for estrogen detoxification.

Thyroid Imbalances

The thyroid gland releases thyroid hormones which are T4 (thyroxine) and T3 (triiodothyronine).

"Low thyroid" can be a number of things, including the thyroid actually secreting less of the hormone, or the thyroid gland could be secreting just the right amounts of the hormone, but it doesn't get converted to the active form of the hormone. If you have low thyroid function, not caused by an autoimmune condition, supplement your diet with selenium, iodine, and tyrosine.

Detoxify your body from heavy metals, especially mercury. If you have the old style mercury fillings, have them removed. Hair mineral analysis helps to pinpoint what minerals and toxins are found in the body (as discussed in chapter 1). We like to help our clients detoxify in a healthy way.

Nutritionist, TV host, Author and speaker, Julie Daniluk recommended dulse also known as sea lettuce or dulse chips. Dulse is dark-red edible seaweed, originating from the east. It tastes great and it is good for the thyroid.

Again, don't underestimate the importance of sleep, as Dr. Tara Andresen, ND says, "If you don't get enough sleep, you end up with an underperforming thyroid." If you have hypothyroidism, Dr. Andrea Maxim, ND suggests a clean diet which would include gluten-free and dairy-free foods because gluten is inflammatory towards the thyroid.

If you have symptoms of both low thyroid and high thyroid function, get tested for Hashimoto's thyroiditis. It is an autoimmune condition whereby your own immune system attacks your thyroid. Julie Daniluk suggests that people with Hashimoto's should look into plant sterols which help modulate the immune system.

Calories vs. Hormones

Dr. Makoto Trotter, ND, said that one of the biggest myths and misconceptions when it comes to fat loss is the "calories in vs. calories out" myth, especially when hormones are involved.

Importance should be placed on hormonal balance rather than calories. When scientists determine how many calories are in a food they burn it in an oven and measure how much heat it produces. A calorie is the amount of energy required to heat up one litre of water by 1 C. There is a little problem - an oven is not a human body. Some people can eat 3,000 calories a day without any problems and others can eat 1,000 calories a day and still put on body fat. I hear you and I know it isn't fair. The truth is, you can count how many calories are going into your mouth, but you cannot determine how much of that is being used as fuel in the body. Likewise, you simply cannot accurately determine how many calories are being expended through exercise.

As much as you try to race the person next to you on the treadmill, the treadmills and other *fitness machines can't determine your fitness level*. Elliptical machines tend to overestimate the amount of calories you burn. The more fit you are, the fewer calories you burn doing the same activities for the same duration. This is why calorie counting can be a very dangerous game because the calorie math rarely adds up.

Registered Holistic Nutritionist, Lori Kennedy pointed out that if you're hungry all the time, you may be exercising too much. She said that another fat-loss misconception is that eating less will cause fat loss. Lori said, "Women in particular believe that when they drop calories, they lose fat faster, but what actually happens is the thyroid slows down and the adrenals tire out."

Briana Santoro, Founder of *The Naked Label* said, "People trying to lose weight view food as the enemy. That's the wrong relationship with food." Calories are not the enemy. The goal is first and foremost to strive to be healthy with proper hormonal balance and in so doing; you will be able to maintain a healthy weight.

Bearing this in mind, I urge you to pay attention to the signals your body is sending you and get the help you need to balance out your hormonal profile so that you can be happy and healthy. Should you need some guidance, take advantage of our Dream Body MAP session offer at the back of the book. (See page 125-126)

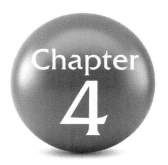

Sleep-
Eat-
Supplement

D id you know that you will spend one-third of your life sleeping? It is an important activity. I often hear, "I need to get more work done, so I sleep less." Think about it for a moment: sleep is more important than the work you are doing because work is work, but *sleep is health*. Your greatest wealth is good health. If you are not sleeping well, you are not being as productive as you could be. You can never really catch up on lost sleep; you can catch up on work, but at what cost?

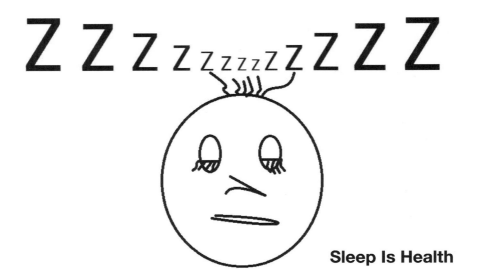

Sleep Is Health

Sleep and Body Transformation

A client who weighed 120 lbs. at five feet eight inches tall needed to gain muscle mass. We worked hard to gain muscle and together we worked up to 132 lbs. On one occasion, when it came to taking his bi-weekly measurements, he had dropped three pounds. He had the opposite problem to most everyone else - he had to fight to gain muscle mass. After this surprising drop, we tried to determine the reason for this loss. His exercise and nutrition regimen had not changed. After much investigation we were able to pinpoint the problem. He had been sleeping 30 minutes less each night. It took us four weeks to gain those precious three pounds, but after only two weeks of less sleep, those pounds rapidly went AWOL. I instructed him to revert back to his previous sleep patterns and as a result he regained the missing pounds.

Another client was an active 73-year-old who was injury prone. These injuries took an inordinate time to heal. As he aged, he started having trouble sleeping. Once we got his sleep on track, old chronic injuries that had lasted months healed in a few weeks.

Good Sleep Critical for Hormone Balance

If you're not sleeping properly, you're not producing enough serotonin. You will likely find that you crave carbohydrates and sweets. Indulging in the munchies will raise serotonin temporarily and then you will experience an inevitable crash and then it becomes a vicious cycle. You can raise serotonin levels in a healthy way by using a combination of supplements (5-HTP) and protein. Serotonin, which is a neurotransmitter, is made from an amino acid called tryptophan. The food that is highest in tryptophan is turkey; that's why you feel sleepy after that Thanksgiving turkey dinner.

If you're not sleeping properly, you have less energy, so you feel the need for stimulants; caffeine and nicotine are the most common. Stimulants will cause cortisol to stay in your blood longer. As a result, you don't have the appropriate amount of energy to put into your workouts even if you can drag yourself off the couch.

Igor Klibanov

Here is an excerpt from the book, *Lights Out: Sleep, Sugar, and Survival,* by T. S. Wiley with Brent Formby, PhD.

"In *Lights Out*, we prove that obesity and the major killers correlated with obesity —heart disease, diabetes, and cancer—are caused by short nights and ridiculously long hours, by literally burning the candle at both ends, and by the electricity that gives us the ability to do it. *The cause is most certainly not overeating fat or a lack of exercise.*"

You can develop insulin resistance while having a perfect diet, but bad sleep. When your hormones are out of balance due to lack of sleep you are putting your health at risk and I don't say this lightly.

During sleep, melatonin is released, which affects all other hormones; there are over 40 different hormones in the body. Melatonin is secreted by a small endocrine gland, the size of a pea, known as the pineal gland - not to be mistaken with the pituitary gland. The release of melatonin is triggered by darkness. It is critical to sleep in a dark room, with absolutely no light whatsoever.

Melatonin and cortisol are antagonistic hormones, meaning that when cortisol is high, melatonin is low. Ideally, your melatonin should be high at bedtime and your cortisol should be low.

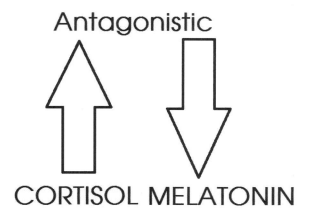

Depression and Anxiety

Poor sleep can lead to depression or anxiety. Serotonin is your happy juice; it is depleted when you lack sleep. This initiates a vicious cycle because you go to your doctor, he or she prescribes antidepressants, and these medications on their own will increase weight without a change in lifestyle or nutrition. One of the side-effects of antidepressant medication is poor sleep and so the cycle continues. What led to the depression in the first place is exacerbated due to the antidepressant medications. There are other side-effects that are not desirable, but that is another topic.

As a result of taking these drugs, certain nutrients are depleted. The most common example of this is using statins (cholesterol-lowering medications). Statins lower co-enzyme Q10 which is a fat-soluble nutrient needed for energy production, among other things. This is known as statin-induced mitochondrial dysfunction. Antidepressants will also deplete chromium, which is needed for blood sugar regulation. In addition, melatonin is depleted which, as you know, is needed to regulate sleep and mood regulation.

Here's some good advice from Caron DeVita, President at Biotics Research Canada: "Don't go completely off meds, it has to be done through the medical doctor." Sam Hannaalla, from Smith's Pharmacy, identified the following medications as those most responsible for fat gain: certain anti-depressants, anti-psychotics, anti-epileptics, diabetic meds (sulfonylurea), corticosteroids, and so on. He suggested emotional support groups for people on antidepressants, which will help lose body fat. Now *that* is pretty progressive thinking for a pharmacist!

Sherry Torkos is a Holistic Pharmacist and author of The Canadian Encyclopedia of Natural Medicine. She shares her wealth of information on the effects of medicines on weight gain:

"There are many drugs that can impact body weight by causing increased appetite, reducing metabolism or causing fluid retention or fatigue. Here are some of the most common ones:

- *Antidepressants such as amitriptyline, paroxetine, and mirtazapine — affects appetite.*

- *Anticonvulsants such as valproic acid — affects appetite and metabolism.*

- *Antipsychotics such as clozapine, chlorpromazine, olanzapine — increases appetite.*

- *Beta-blockers (used for lowering blood pressure and regulating heart rate) such as atenolol, metoprolol and propranolol can cause fatigue and reduced metabolism.*

- *Birth control pills and the Depo Provera injection can affect both appetite and metabolism and cause weight gain in some women.*

- *Corticosteroids such as prednisone (when taken for long periods of time) cause weight gain, particularly around the mid-section by reducing metabolism and increasing appetite.*

- *Glyburide (a drug used for Type 2 diabetes) — increases appetite.*

- *Lithium, a drug used for bipolar disorder/manic — depression can affect appetite.*

Sherry Torkos suggested you take these steps to prevent or reverse these side-effects:

- *Increase exercise and activity level to keep metabolism working efficiently.*

- *Choose healthy, satisfying, low-calorie snacks such as vegetables, yogurt, and seeds.*

- *Talk to your doctor or pharmacist about whether there is an alternative therapy to treat your condition.*

Neutralize Adverse Side-Effects

Hair mineral analysis can identify which nutrients have been depleted as a result of taking medications. We then supplement in order to help counteract the effects of medication-induced weight gain. In my experience as a fitness professional, this is a very difficult process. If you go to a personal trainer who is not aware of these things, you will be told to workout harder. If your body chemistry is out of whack, no amount of exercise is going to fix it. It is important to plug the holes that medications create.

Cortisol increases with poor sleep. We discussed cortisol earlier at length and so I will not rehash cortisol facts. Suffice it to say that this is an important factor which affects body transformation. Managing stress is one of the best things you can do to counteract the rise in cortisol.

This quiz is a tool to determine whether lack of quality sleep is sabotaging fat loss efforts. I encourage clients to have sleep habits that support their body transformation goals.

The Sleep Quiz

Do you go to bed after 11 p.m.?

Do you wake up before 6 a.m.?

Does it take more than 10 minutes to fall asleep?

Do you wake up throughout the night (including washroom visits)?

Do you take any medications to help you sleep?

Are there any lights in your room (moonlight, bright neon lights on an alarm clock, etcetera)?

Do you keep any electronics beside your bed?

Do you use an alarm clock to wake up?

When you wake up, do you feel refreshed, or tired?

First take the test for yourself and then let's take a closer look. Ideally you should aim to be in bed before 11 p.m. and schedule your life to allow undisturbed sleep until after 6 a.m.. This is the suggested minimum hours you should sleep. If you want to go to bed before 11 p.m. and wake up after 6 a.m., I highly recommend it. You should fall asleep relatively quickly at night and should sleep all the way through. If you get up or wake up and fall back to sleep immediately you are still experiencing disturbed sleep which is not optimal.

Don't drink liquids close to bedtime so that you will not need to go to the washroom. If you stop drinking liquids at 6 p.m. and still wake up to go to the washroom, you may have an underlying problem and I suggest you talk to your physician. Black out all lights, including LED lighting and remove electronic devices such as cell phones, iPads, and laptops.

Ideally, if your sleep patterns are set up as they should, you should wake up before the alarm clock goes off. The rude awakening the alarm clock gives the body causes a stress reaction and you release cortisol right off the bat. Not a good way to start the day. It is much better to wake up naturally and you will feel more refreshed and ready to take on the day. Now is your chance to throw that noisy alarm clock against the wall, go ahead! There is something called a natural alarm clock and I don't mean your dog. It is an alarm clock that gradually emits light and assimilates sunrise.

Normal brainwave activity is disturbed when you keep your cellphone next to your bed and this interferes with your sleep. The world will not fall apart if you don't check your texts and messages before bed; it can wait until morning. Your health and sleep are more important. I am not alone in saying this. Dr. Makoto Trotter, ND says, "Another big problem is using electronic devices before bed, and that throws off the melatonin."

You should not require medications to fall asleep. Melatonin supplements are a temporal support and should not be used for extended periods of time. Once you have reestablished your sleep cycle you should stop taking supplements.

Charles Poliquin suggests you sleep "in a cave." Even the smallest amount of light can upset your body's' circadian rhythms, which follow a 24-hour cycle, responding primarily to light and darkness in your environment. This cycle affects cortisol, serotonin, and melatonin levels. Interestingly enough, abnormal circadian rhythms have been associated with obesity, depression, diabetes, bipolar, and seasonal affective disorder.

Charles Poliquin says that you can wake someone up by shining a flashlight on their feet. Give it a try!

Strategies for Better Sleep

Nothing drives your cortisol levels up faster than stress. Don't have a fight with your significant other before you go to sleep and if you do, make up! Never go to sleep angry.

Ensure that you have proper sleep hygiene. What does that mean? It means that your bedroom should not be used as an office or television room. There are only *two things* for which you should use your bedroom, and they are, frankly, sleep and sex.

Igor Klibanov

I know you don't want to hear this, but you should not be on your laptop or ipad in bed. In addition to keeping your bedroom for the two aforementioned activities only, you should keep your bedroom cool. Research points to room temperature playing a part in SIDS (Sudden Infant Death Syndrome). For adults, an optimal temperature in the bedroom should be between 18 C to 20 C.

Turkey and Tomatoes

My first strategy with my clients is supplementation, but if clients are distrustful of those, then I suggest they eat turkey and tomatoes for dinner. You can have other foods with it, but make sure your get those two foods in. My insomniac grandmother tried it upon my recommendation and it worked for her. Turkey contains tryptophan, which gets converted to serotonin, which in turn gets converted to melatonin. Tomatoes contain straight up melatonin.

Rakowski's Sleep Window

What would be your ideal sleep window? Say, between 11 p.m. and 7 a.m.? Yours may differ. How many hours do you *actually* sleep? Robert Rakowski is a chiropractor, kinesiologist, and Certified Clinical Nutritionist in Houston, Tex. He implements a regimen whereby clients sleep only those hours that they actually remain asleep and no longer. Then upon waking, they stay awake for the rest of the day while not taking stimulants or naps. On the second night the amount of sleep can be increased by 15 minutes on each end of the set time. Rakowsi claims that within a week he can get people who have been sleeping three hours a night to sleep eight hours a night.

My theory is that taking a person who is sleep deprived, depriving them even more for one night stimulates a reverse response.

Melatonin

Not everyone has the same kind of issues when it comes to sleep. Some have trouble falling asleep; some have trouble staying asleep. Some people have both and they will tell you how it wears them down.

Taking melatonin supplements is not 100 percent reliable. You will need to use the supplement for two weeks in order to gauge if it works for you. It is good, therefore, to combine strategies and you can stack these things together because certain supplements are good for those who have a hard time falling asleep, while others address different issues, such as staying asleep. Dr. Tara Andresen, ND suggests, "If you are having trouble staying asleep, try slow-release melatonin."

5-HTP (5 – hydroxytryptophan)

5-HTP is a precursor to melatonin and an amino acid and chemical compound, naturally produced in your

Igor Klibanov

body as it makes serotonin. Serotonin regulates your mood, appetite, sleep, libido, and body temperature. *A word of caution: 5-HTP is not to be used while taking antidepressants. Taking 5-HTP with medications used for depression might cause serious side-effects including heart problems, shivering, and anxiety. Please consult your doctor.*

Limit the 4 Cs

Limit your intake of the 4 Cs: caffeine, cigarettes, coffee, and chocolate as well as your intake of alcohol.

Journaling Your Thoughts

If your mind is racing and you are thinking about all you have to do the next day, write out a list and leave your worries on that paper. Write down things for which you are grateful or a good thing that happened during the day. Journaling your thoughts and feelings can be therapeutic and an effective tool in calming the mind.

Now that you know more about how sleep affects your health, take the steps necessary to improve your sleep. Guard your sleep time and make it count; you are worth it after all. Remember: Sleep is health!

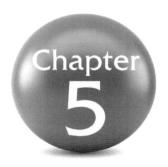

Chapter 5

Plan to Progress

W hat is your goal? Do you want to run a 10 km, do you want to have more energy, or do you want to look like Victoria Secret's latest supermodel, Candice Swanepoel? You can't progress if you don't know where you are headed. It is like getting on the subway without a destination in mind.

Measure What Is Relevant to Your Goal

If your goal is to look a certain way then what the scale says is irrelevant and you will use the mirror as your guide. Take before-and-after pictures as well as progress pictures along the way. Use body fat or skin-fold measurements as a guide as to whether you are moving in the right direction. If you think about it, the number on the scale does not matter as long as you are progressing towards looking the way you want to look, based on your goals.

Dr. Andreo Spina, an excellent chiropractor said, "People have the illusion of homeostasis. The truth is you're either deteriorating or building."

You must quantify. If you want to run 10 km, it is irrelevant how many pushups you can do. Keep your eyes on the prize.

Take the First Steps to Looking AND Feeling Better for FREE!

www.fitnesssolutionsplus.ca

Train Hard!

Train hard relative to your abilities. That does not mean that everybody should lift extremely heavy weights or run long distances, but you should lift weights relative to your abilities. Bear in mind your abilities improve quickly as a beginner. What you are doing in the gym today should not be the same thing a month from now. The more of a beginner you are, and the more deconditioned you are, the faster you will see results. For this reason, don't be afraid to increase your weights at every workout or increase the number of repetitions you do in a set. Your goal should be to make progress at each workout and there are many ways to do that.

One of the biggest mistakes people make is to underestimate their abilities and their strength.

I see women using pink dumbbells and they do triceps kickbacks because they are afraid if they lift anything heavier they will bulk up. This is not true! You will *not* end up looking like Arnold Schwarzenegger.

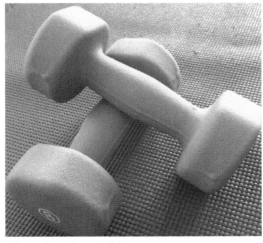

Photo by: Jewel Fries

75

Multi-Joint Exercises

Use primarily multi-joint exercises such as pushups which use both elbow and shoulder joints together, and squats use the ankle, knee, and hip —all together. A single-joint exercise, for example, is a biceps curl. Use primarily, but not entirely multi-joint exercise; do roughly 80 percent multi-joint exercises and 20 percent single-joint exercises.

Multi-joint exercises use many muscles at the same time. Squats use your quadriceps (front of the thighs), hamstrings (backs of the thighs), gluteus maximus (buttocks), and if you are using a bar it will also work your abdominals (stomach muscles) and your lower back. That is five muscles in one exercise, whereas if you were to do separate exercises to work the same muscles, it would take more time. This kind of exercise will speed up your metabolism so much more than doing individual exercises.

Balance Out Any Muscle Imbalances

This is critical and we will have a chapter dedicated to this subject alone. Everyone has muscle imbalances, the most common of which are caused by bad posture. Tight chest means that you likely have weak back muscles. If you have an exaggerated lower back curvature you will likely suffer from pain due to a tight lower back and weak abdominals together with tight hip flexors. If you have rounded shoulders, abstain from doing chest exercises until you have balanced out your muscles. Only do exercises that reverse the imbalances and then once that has been addressed, continue with chest exercises on a 1:1 ratio. If you are not sure what your imbalances are, come and see one of our trainers, and we can identify them (take advantage of the FREE gift on page 127).

Full range of motion means full anatomical range of motion. What may be full range of motion for one may not be for another. Generally speaking, women have a better range of motion because their joints are not as tight as men. Using full range of motion guarantees that you not only gain strength, but also flexibility. That's right. You get more flexible with strength training when it is done properly.

Put Effort Into It

Bump up the effort, unless you have adrenal fatigue, as already discussed. And if you do, put as much effort into it as needed to stay motivated. Most women underestimate their strength.

If your exercise hurts your joints, don't do it. The saying, "No pain, no gain" is out the window – *that* saying applies to muscles and not joints! If you feel the discomfort of muscular exertion that is one thing, but the moment you feel pain in your joints, even if you *suspect* you might feel pain in the joints, STOP what you are doing immediately!

Igor Klibanov

For God's Sake, DON'T Use Balance Implements

This means don't stand on BOSU balls unless you are in the circus! Please, don't use balance implements unless you are involved in rehabilitation. I see a number of people using unstable implements for balance exercises improperly *without reasonable justification.*

Balance apparatus activates, but *does not strengthen the core*. Let me explain: if you pick up any exercise physiology textbook, you will learn that to increase strength in a muscle, you have to contract with at least 40 percent of that muscle's maximal voluntary contraction. When you are standing on a balance board or ball doing your best seal impersonation you are only contracting with up to 10 percent. You are not getting anywhere near the threshold necessary to obtain strengthening effects. This is only applies if you are a beginner. When you are advanced it takes 70 – 80 percent maximum voluntary contraction to achieve strengthening results, so the 40 percent will no longer work for the advanced weight lifter.

When you do a regular standing biceps curl, the first muscle to contract is the calf muscle in order to stabilize you. Let's say you are lifting 10-lb. dumb bells in each hand; now the front of the body has 20 lbs. more weight than the back of your body and the muscles that prevent you from tipping over are your calves. Do you expect to attain strong calves from doing bicep curls? No! Likewise doing curls on a stability ball will not make your core stronger.

Your body has three primary types of muscle fibers: slow-twitch, fast-twitch A, and fast-twitch X. Here is a simplified explanation: the fast-twitch fibers are responsible for speed, strength, and power, and the slow-twitch fibers are responsible for endurance. An exercise physiology textbook will tell you that the threshold for engaging the fast-twitch fibers is 40 percent (for fast-twitch A) and 70 percent (for fast-twitch X) of your maximal voluntary contraction. And when you're doing balance exercises on an unstable implement, you're not using anywhere near that much.

Some argue that balance apparatus training will improve your balance. Unless you are thinking of enrolling in the latest Cirque Du Soleil show, how much balancing do you need to do on a daily basis? Yes, your balance will improve, but does it improve balance in a way that carries over to everyday life? Life happens on stable ground unless you're a skateboarder, snowboarder, surfer, and so on, in which case, there is certainly a reason to use unstable implements. If you want to improve your balance, wouldn't it make sense to train in the way you actually live?

You might think that there's a carry-over from doing balance exercises on unstable surfaces to stable surfaces. It's only logical but, unfortunately, that's not the case. The body has two reflexes responsible for balance: righting reflexes and equilibrium reflexes. Righting reflexes are responsible for restoring your balance when you're moving over solid ground. Equilibrium reflexes are responsible for restoring your balance when you're moving over unstable surfaces (for example, standing on a moving bus, skateboarding, or snowboarding). The neurological mechanisms that govern each one are vastly different, so there is minimal carry-over from one to the other.

The argument goes that since doing balance exercises on unstable surfaces engages more muscles -and let's not forget that "engages" does not mean "strengthens" -, it burns more calories. There's some truth to that but think about it: can you lift more weight, and do more reps on a stable or an unstable surface? Of course you can lift more weight and perform more repetitions on a stable surface. By using more weight and more repetitions on a stable surface, you'll burn more calories than using lighter weights and fewer repetitions on an unstable surface.

By now you know that "engages" doesn't mean "strengthens." Let's say for a second that it does engage the stabilizer muscles (which it does). So what? What benefit will it have? In a healthy person, there is no additional benefit. In a person with some sort of prior dysfunction around a joint where the stabilizer muscles are "sleeping" —only then does it start to have benefits —in retraining the stabilizers to engage.

Now is all of this to say that balance exercises on an unstable surface are useless? No, far from it. There is a time and a place to use unstable surfaces, but it *must be justified*. One of the correct ways to use balance exercises on unstable surfaces is in rehabilitation scenarios where certain stabilizers have "fallen asleep" as a result of prior injury.

Excessive and Exclusive

Cardiovascular Exercise Can Make You Fat

Excessive and exclusive cardiovascular exercise burns muscle. Each pound of muscle you have burns about 13 calories a day (at bed rest), which does not sound like much, but imagine losing 10 lbs. of muscle. So even if you have a desk job you are burning way more calories than if you were at rest. It adds up. If you lose muscle, you are burning fewer calories a day when in fact you want to burn *more* calories a day (within reason).

Fuel efficiency sounds good if you are a car or an endurance athlete, but it is *not good* if you want to be lean.

Igor Klibanov

The more efficient your body gets, the fewer calories are burned and again, you want to burn more calories, not less. Does this mean you should never do cardiovascular exercise? No, that is not what I am saying. Do running or swimming in conjunction with strength training. Strength training will speed up fat loss. Keep your cardiovascular exercise under 30 minutes.

When I do public speaking engagements I often show a photo of a well-known endurance athlete and ask the audience to guess the woman's age. Without fail they guess 15 – 20 years older than the actual age of the athlete. Although she is a long-endurance athlete and is fit, she looks much older than her actual age. As I have said before, excessive cardio ages you; it stimulates excess cortisol.

Stretching

Only stretch what *needs* to be stretched. Often people have a habit of stretching everything and that is not a good habit because different muscles have different optimal lengths. Furthermore, different people have different optimal lengths for the same muscles. A gymnast will need much more shoulder flexibility than a computer geek.

I learned from Pavel Tsatsouline that you need to give your body strength as well as length. Typically, people who naturally want to stretch because they enjoy it are already flexible to begin with. You naturally gravitate to what you are good at; if you are naturally flexible you should probably do more strength training. If you are naturally drawn to strength training, chances are you need more flexibility. This subject is impossible to explain without going into technical jargon and since I can't insert a video into a book format, I suggest talking to a professional about what and how you should stretch, based on your individual needs.

Jana Webb said that one of the biggest misconceptions when it comes to stretching and yoga is that people need to be super flexible and that stretching needs to be intense to be effective.

Kareen Hodgins said that the biggest misconception she sees when it comes to stretching and yoga is that when you're stretching, you have to go all the way. No you don't. In her yoga practice she noted that another misconception is that you have to make the body fit the pose. "Not the case," she says. "You need to make the pose fit the body. Modify, adjust and use props. You don't have to be a supermodel or super skinny to do yoga. Any size and shape can and should do yoga."

Mabel Pun said that in her experience the biggest misconception when it comes to stretching and yoga is that you need to push hard. "If you do that," she said, "the muscle shortens. To truly lengthen, the muscle needs to relax." Another misconception she noted was, "If you can stretch like a pretzel, it must be a good stretch." She said, "Not true. We all have different bone structures."

Some think that static stretching is *bad* for you and some argue that it is in fact *good* for you. The truth is somewhere in the middle. Again, stretching when done correctly can strengthen muscles, but when it is done unnecessarily it can weaken muscles.

Dr. Allan Austin, DC, has this to say about stretching: "You cannot stretch a muscle. You can functionally lengthen, but not structurally. According to my mother - and I agree with her - 'nature knows best.'" The only animals that stretch are cats, and that's not static; that's dynamic. Animals don't stretch after they workout, and certainly not before working out. Race horses don't do it. Warm up and warm down. Don't stretch."

Jason Helman, from *Jason Helman Golf* admitted, "I've gotten away from stretching. When I didn't stretch, I always seemed to play better." Jason suggested limiting stretching to loosening anything that feels tight that particular day. Considering that it's coming from one of Canada's top golfing instructors, you should probably listen.

The Scale

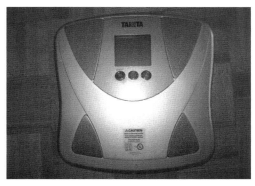

Bathroom scales are great for measuring hydration, but awful for measuring body fat. Leading up to my powerlifting competitions I use the scale twice a day to ensure that I am on track for making the weight category for my weight class. It was not a reflection of my muscle or fat status, but rather a reflection of my hydration status. That is an appropriate use of a scale. For people who are on diuretic medications that regulate blood pressure and water retention and such, the scale becomes a valuable tool to monitor hydration levels.

Bathroom scales are not a suitable gauge of body fat because weight consists of more than just fat. It consists of water, muscle, bones, blood, skin, and much more. I don't think anyone would be happy to lose a leg, even though that is a method of weight loss, and so, to use the scale for body fat is not appropriate.

Are You Planning to Progress?

In conclusion, most people go about exercising the wrong way, and are not putting in enough effort and progressing the way they should. They go to the gym and do the same workout year after year and expect different results. They are afraid to lift heavier weights. Some blame their age, the truth is that the older and weaker you are, the more you stand to benefit from strength training.

Make sure you are progressing in your workouts. People who benefit the most from exercise are *not* the elite athletes, but the frail and the elderly. If they have not taken care of themselves over the years, they have lost much strength and muscle mass. They stand to gain the most with the least amount of effort. They regain their strength back faster than someone who has been training for years. The more deconditioned you are the faster you are able to progress, whereas an elite athlete has to train for years to better their personal best performances by milliseconds. In short, *keep challenging yourself!*

There should *not* be pink dumbbells in a gym! I don't know why they exist. Your body does not know if the dumbbells are pink or chrome. Alright, I will now climb down from my soap box.

Don't make the mistake of not listening to your body. Adjust your exercise to your own unique body. Your fitness program needs to be adjusted, based on your *own* goals and your *own* body type. A significant mistake is to exercise without the guidance of a professional, because not only can they guide and motivate you, they can educate you. Save yourself years of trial and error. Your personal trainer will share their training and experience with you so that you don't have to take years figuring it all out by yourself, and possibly injuring yourself along the way.

A workout does not have to be an hour long, so the "all-or-nothing" mentality prevails. You think that since you can't do an hour every day, then you just will skip your workout altogether. Ten minutes of exercise of strength training is better than none! You can squeeze a few squats in between commercials while watching television. You don't have to go to the gym or get changed. Just do squats at every break and you will speed up your metabolism and improve your blood sugar handling and improve your muscle tone. As I have said before, a short workout is better than nothing.

Consistency is key when it comes to exercise. As Mike Otani says, "You have to shower anyway, and you might as well go to the gym and shower there. And since you're already at the gym, you might as well get in a few minutes of exercise." Whatever you are doing, make sure you *measure your progress* and you must *plan to progress*: if you are not assessing, you are guessing.

Take the First Steps to Looking
AND Feeling Better for FREE!

www.fitnesssolutionsplus.ca

Chapter 6

Stand up Straight!

Stand up straight and tall; it's not just a matter of aesthetics, it is also about efficiency. A well-aligned human being is a marvelous piece of architecture because it is an intricate design of bone stacked upon bone, which takes little energy to hold upright. Take a look at your own unique body structure. If you lean forward, your neck and lower back muscles must contract to prevent you from tipping over. If these muscles are in a constant state of contraction, they are cutting off blood flow to other muscles and organs.

Posture can cause problems seemingly unrelated to muscles and joints such as migraines, digestive dysfunction, sexual dysfunction, and more. When any part of the musculoskeletal system is out of alignment, this is where the above-mentioned problems come in as well as shoulder pain and lower back issues, which you might expect.

Good Posture for More than Just Looks

Your posture affects more than just your aesthetics. The farther forward your head travels, the less the blood flow to your brain and, the greater the risk of migraines and stroke. Never mind poor concentration, watery eyes, bags under your eyes, and other problems. Bad posture also saps your endurance. You use minimal muscle force to move around if you have good posture. When you are out of alignment, you use more muscle force just to live and wonder why you don't have much energy to get through the day. I could go on about the effects of bad and good posture on your digestion, on your reproductive organs, your joints, and more, but let's get to the good stuff: Fixing it.

Aside from causing you to look like you lost a few pounds, standing straight and tall has many benefits, including injury prevention. Kelly Starrett said, "If you don't want to get injured, wrap yourself in a bubble suit." That may be true. It gives even more importance to conscious injury prevention.

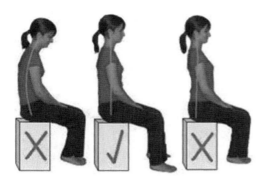

Injury Prevention

If you're injury prone, one of the culprits may be poor posture. Muscles work like a finely-tuned symphony. Even in a simple movement like walking, or reaching for something in the cupboard, muscles contract with a certain sequence and force. Your brain controls this sequence of muscular contractions in order for you to have correct co-ordination and motor control skills necessary to complete the task. When you have tuned up the symphony, the right muscles will be firing with the right amount of force at the right time. Dancers have advanced co-ordination and motor control skills — not that I would know, *since I don't dance*. It is purely an observation! I do, however, listen to the band Modern Talking, and so should you. But I digress.

Poor posture will affect the sequence and force of every movement. If that happens, you're more likely to get injured and develop arthritis. Let's look at the motion necessary to take a step. Whenever you walk, or take a step, there is a particular sequence of muscular contractions starting with the foot muscles, then the calf, followed by the muscles behind the knee, then the hamstrings and glutes, transferring to the opposite lower back and then opposite upper back. This is the sequence on the back side of your body; there is a different sequence for the opposing muscles on the front. When this sequence is altered, the result is variation in gait.

Ladies, take note that wearing high heels will throw the sequence off too. Men, don't think you get off lightly, since poor posture can throw off this sequence too. When you see someone walking with an exaggerated sway of the hips (and it is not because they are wearing heels) it is caused by a weak gluteus medius, which in turn puts you at risk for knee problems such as ACL and MCL tears. In case you are curious, there are three glutes: Gluteus maximus, gluteus medius, and gluteus minimus.

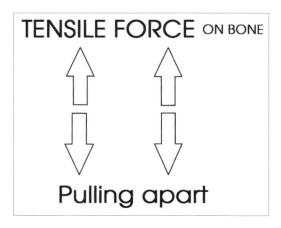

There are three kinds of forces the joints are exposed to in the body: Tensile force, (it acts to pull the joints apart), shear force (sliding gliding or rubbing), and compressive force (like pushing down on, gravity or weight).

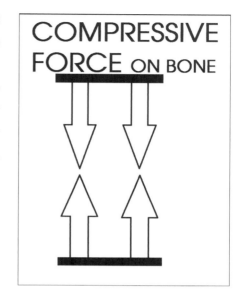

Shearing forces are unaligned forces pushing one part of a body in one direction, and another part of the body in the opposite direction. Joints are able to contend with tensile and compressive forces, but are not made for shearing friction or rubbing together. The ACL (anterior cruciate ligament) is meant to prevent shear force across the knee joint. When the muscular sequence is off and your gait is affected, rubbing of the joints occurs which causes tears in the ligament. The same thing happens with the MCL (medial collateral ligament).

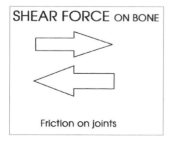

While we do extensive biomechanical testing with our clients to identify their imbalances, it's not practical to do so in a book format. A rudimentary explanation is this: if you have an exaggerated lower-back curve (swayback), flatten it; if you have a flat back (hunchback), create a curve there. The simple test involves standing with your back to the wall and noting the three points of contact and how much space there is between the lower back and the wall. If you can slide your hand right through the curve of your back and the wall, you have an exaggerated curvature of the spine. Ideally you should only be able to slide half your flat hand behind your back.

Go take a look in the mirror. Don't change anything don't fix anything, - just look in the mirror. Are your shoulders slumped forward? Now stand sideways. Do you have an exaggerated upper-back curve? Is your head really far ahead of your shoulders? In the past, have you actively tried to correct your bad posture, but failed miserably? It helps to have someone take pictures of you in minimal clothing, and analyze them.

Habit vs. Conditioning

Chiropractor, Dr. Andreo Spina says that posture is 95 percent habit and five percent conditioning. I agree with this. You can do all the posture exercises, but really you have to *form a habit*. Dr. Spina's suggestion is to set up reminders: buy little red stickers, and post them anywhere. He said, "Injury prevention should be a side-effect of good mobility and good strength." What we do with clients is to ask them to set a reminder in their electronic gadgets to every hour and when the alarm goes off they are to check their posture and maintain their self-awareness.

Martin Reader and Ryan Caicco suggest that you make sure your shoulders sit on a properly stabilized pelvis — awareness is key. For issues related to posture, they take a four-pronged approach and address these four areas:

Loosening your hip flexors.
Strengthening glutes.
Mobilizing the thoracic spine.
Reinforcing overhead patterns.

Movement Specialist, Dewey Nielsen said that the biggest movement problems he sees in the sedentary, middle-aged population are thoracic spine issues, stiff hips, and lower-back problems. In my experience, good posture will take four to six months to create, depending on how bad posture was to begin with. Kelly Starrett suggests that if you have hypermobility, you should create stability using the muscular system, not bone-on-bone. If you have bad posture, both conditioning *and* establishing good habits are important.

Two Key ingredients to help correct posture are:

1. *Frequency*

2. *Force*

Igor Klibanov

Frequency of exercise is absolutely necessary in order to achieve good posture. In other words, you must do posture exercises with extremely high frequency - 15-30 times a day or more. The nice thing is that these exercises take 60 seconds or less, and do not require equipment.

Do your posture exercises when you're driving or at a red light. Red lights last 60 seconds or more which is a perfect opportunity to practice your posture exercises. If you have the "pleasure" of driving during rush hour, you're stationary more than you're driving which is an excellent opportunity to spend even more time working to improve your posture without taking much time out of your day.

Force is key to improving posture. When I say, "force", I mean the magnitude of the strength of the contraction of the muscle. Even if you do 30 minutes of exercise, spread throughout the day; that still leaves 23.5 hours spent *not* doing those exercises.

How then, do you change your posture? Make those 30 minutes have substantially higher force than the other 23.5 hours. Let's do some math: At rest, most muscles contract with one to two percent of their maximal force. This is an involuntary state of contraction, which you need just to give you structure. To counterbalance that, those 30 minutes of posture training you do must have substantially higher force. We know from sport science that you can hold a contraction with 50-60 percent of your maximal force for 60-120 seconds (depending on the muscle group). We then know that whenever you do your posture exercises, squeeze your muscles with 50-60 percent of your maximal force to counterbalance the other 23.5 hours of low force.

Posture exercises should be done daily. I have purposely not talked about specific exercises for posture. The reason is that bad posture can be caused by many different things —you can have a hunchback or a swayback. You might have scoliosis. You can have rotation of the hips. Giving blanket exercises would improve posture in some, and make it worse in others. If you'd like an examination of your particular posture and a specific exercise recommendation for your body, that's a service our trainers offer.

Improper Breathing Can Cause Tightness

Posture and breath awareness go hand in hand. If you are slouched over your desk for hours at work, you will not be breathing the way you should. Here's a little test to do while sitting right at your desk or at the dining room table:

Put one hand on your chest and one hand on your belly and just breathe naturally. Which hand moves more? The one on the chest or belly? Don't read any further; it's very important that you do this test without knowing what we're looking for, so do it now. I'll wait.

If you're breathing into your belly, pat yourself on the back. That's the way you should be breathing. If you find yourself breathing into your chest, you may be setting yourself up for a host of problems.

Do you feel chronic tightness in your body? Is it in your neck, shoulders, lower back or hamstrings? Do you have a constant urge to stretch the muscles that feel tight? If you do stretch them, chances are you feel temporary relief, and then a few hours or even minutes later, those areas continue to feel tight. The underlying cause of your tightness, believe it or not, is due to faulty breathing mechanics.

Here is a simple test to illustrate what I mean: Put one hand on your neck. Now take a deep breath into your chest (on purpose). What do you feel your neck muscles doing when you inhale into the chest? Chances are you feel those muscles contract or shorten. Now repeat the test, but breathe into the belly; take a normal breath, not an exaggerated one. Now what do you feel in your neck? Chances are you feel nothing. The muscle tension there doesn't really change.

The neck is just an example, but the same reactions happen in the muscles of the chest, the shoulders, the lower back and even the hamstrings.

If you consistently breathe into the chest, those muscles chronically shorten, and you get a feeling of stiffness. You can stretch your tight muscles until the cows come home, but until you correct your breathing, any corrective efforts will be useless.

In addition to tightness of the muscles, poor breathing can sap your energy. If you breathe properly (that means breathing into your belly, not your chest, and breathing 12 times a minute or fewer), you oxygenate your tissues very well. Ironically, *the more you breathe, the less oxygen you have* (the rationale for this is a bit too long to explain. If you're curious, look up the "Bohr effect.") So once your breathing has been corrected, that's another energy zapper gone.

Other Effects of Poor Breathing

Here are other effects of faulty breathing mechanics:

- *Lower back pain*

- *Fat loss resistance*

- *Poor endurance*

- *Low energy throughout the day*

- *Digestive problems*

Igor Klibanov

How Can I Correct Faulty Breathing Mechanics?

The solution is fairly simple. Lie down for five minutes. This can be done first thing when waking up, or as you are lying in bed before you fall asleep. Put one hand on the belly and the other hand on your chest. Simply focus on making the hand on the belly move and keep the hand on the chest as steady as possible. This drill should be done every day, ideally twice a day for at least three weeks. By then, you should naturally be breathing into your stomach. It helps if you set little reminders for yourself throughout the day. Set up a little message on your smartphone that prompts you at regular intervals to check your breathing.

In conclusion, self-awareness is key. Learn to carry yourself with confidence, with correct posture and proper breathing and you will feel the benefits. Increased posture is one of the best ways to improve your confidence. Stand up straight, take a deep breath and you'll be doing both your body and mind a favour.

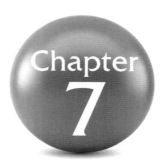

Chapter 7

Time

There's no such thing as lack of time. What we need to address here is a matter of priority. Ask yourself: "Is exercise and health on my priority list?" Most people brush their teeth in the morning regardless of what is going on in their lives. Exercise should be the same — an automatic and non-negotiable part of your day. Bill Gates, with his billions of dollars, has the same 24 hours you have. If your physical health and fitness are low on your priority list, you will not be motivated to pursue these goals either. Best intentions are not enough.

Make Exercising and Eating Right a Priority

Find a strong enough reason to take care of yourself. At some point you have to realize that *you are worth it* and actually believe it. One of Sean Croxton's strategies for staying motivated in your exercise and nutrition is to *have a big enough reason to do it.* He says that it is important to know what your "why" is. Sean, who is the creator of *Underground Wellness* says, "Often, this may have to do with things that are outside of you (like looking good for a party or the beach, and so on). Better to focus on how it will impact you and your relationships.

Would you feel better? Would you have better relationships with your kids or spouse? Would you be able to travel easier?" We will discuss motivation in more detail in the next chapter, but when I asked Sean what he would say to the busy CEO or stay-at-home mom who says he or she doesn't have time to exercise and eat right, his answer was, "Make time. If it's important enough, you will do it. Leo Tolstoy had 13 kids when he wrote *War and Peace.*"

When I asked personal trainer, Bruce Krahn the same question, he said something similar: "We're all busy. It's not a matter of time, but a matter of priority. Barack Obama works out six days a week." When it comes to staying motivated, Bruce pointed out the reasons why some struggle: "Their goals do not excite them enough to keep them going.

You have to be heavily, emotionally invested. If you don't have that emotional investment, get mentors who've achieved what you'd like to achieve. Hang out with them and it rubs off on you."

Bruce's advice was, "Don't suffer from paralysis by analysis. Make a decision and follow through." He also warned, "Don't get distracted by shiny objects. Stick to fundamentals. They remain the same, regardless of the program."

How should you eat and exercise if you have a desk job?

It is important to work within your time restraints and do what you can, given the environment you live and work in. Most of us are in a desk job unless we have really cool jobs, like entrepreneurs or personal trainers.

While desk jobs may be good for our bank accounts, they aren't doing our health any favours. I know what you're thinking: "I exercise for an hour four to six days a week." That's wonderful, and I encourage you to keep it up. However, even exercising for an hour a day doesn't offset sitting on your butt for 15 hours a day. Sorry.

I asked Toronto chiropractor, Dr. Brian Dower, what the biggest ergonomic mistakes people make were and his answer was simply, "Too much sitting." He suggested that this was the cause of hip flexors shortening, back injuries, and shoulder tension. He pointed out that most work environments are made for someone who is five feet 10 inches. Some of us are not that tall, and some of us are taller. He suggested you do some chin tucks while sitting at your desk to alleviate neck strain.

While we can suggest fancy ergonomic devices when we go into offices for ergonomic assessments, what produces the best results is simply getting up and walking around every 20 – 30 minutes. The quip I often hear is, "But I'm too busy for that. My job is important." Stop your whining! Isn't your health more important than your job?

Here's how you automatically build a short walk into your day: First thing you do when you arrive at work is drink two glasses of water. Soon enough, you'll feel the need to go to the washroom. There's your walk built right into your day. When you come back to your desk, drink another glass of water. Again, soon enough, you'll be going to the washroom. Simple? You bet. What can you expect as a result of implementing this win-win strategy? Besides staying well-hydrated, you will benefit by having:

- *More energy*
- *Less lower back pain*
- *Less eye strain*
- *Less stress*
- *Maybe even fat loss*

Now let's talk nutrition for a desk jockey. You know the saying, "Out of sight, out of mind"? The opposite is true too. If it's within your line of sight, *it will get eaten*. If you have chocolate bars stashed in your desk, they'll get eaten — no matter how strong your willpower. If you have a bowl full of veggies within arms' reach at all times, they'll get eaten too, and you will not have to pay much attention to it.

This simple strategy alone has been responsible for the loss of dozens of pounds for our clients. And, constantly snacking on vegetables throughout the day makes it that much easier to resist (or at the very least, moderate) surprise office parties. You know, when that pizza or that birthday cake just assaults you and shoves itself down your throat —you know you've been an innocent victim of this. I was recently asked, "What do you suggest for those who work long hours, don't have time to exercise in the morning, and are too exhausted to exercise by the time they get home at night?" I'm sure that sometimes you feel that way too.

My suggestion don't exercise, sit at home on the couch with a beer in your hand, watch a nice relaxing football game, and have some chips. Just kidding!

Let's address the energy part first. We need to *plug the energy leaks* first, before we start adding in energy.

Igor Klibanov

There are three major energy zappers:

1. *Poor nutrition.*

2. *Poor posture as discussed in the previous chapter.*

3. *Poor breathing patterns as discussed in the previous chapter.*

This chapter isn't about nutrition, but the basics are simple: Eat more vegetables.

Eat one to three servings of meat, fish, or seafood a day. Have so*me healthy fats*, like fatty fish, nuts, seeds, olive oil, coconut oil, and so on. Just doing these things alone will improve your energy.

When a person's posture starts to deviate from "optimal", you require more and more muscular effort to maintain your posture, as discussed in the previous chapter. If your posture is off, you will feel sapped of energy.

Another energy zapper is poor breathing patterns. We discussed this in detail in the previous chapter. Now that your energy leaks are plugged, you can start adding in energy. Exercise is a great way to do that. Again, get rid of the idea that exercise must be an hour long. Do just five minutes of exercise, wherever you can fit it in. Even if you intend on only doing a few minutes, you might find that once you get started, you inevitably end up doing more than you expected. So just get started!

As contradictory as it may seem, exercise is an excellent way to clear away fatigue because when you start exercising, adrenaline starts pumping. Nothing gets rid of fatigue like adrenaline. After you're finished exercising - even if only for five minute , endorphins take over from adrenaline. These are pain-killing hormones that stimulate your brain's pleasure and confidence centers.

What You Can Do Without Weights

Sometimes you'll find you have no equipment and are short on time. This might happen if you travel regularly. My suggestion is that you shorten your workout and you improvise. No skipping workouts!

What can you do? The answer is not as simple as it seems because of *individualization.* Your level of fitness, your age, your goals, and your time will all dictate what exercises you should do. Would it make any sense to give the same exercises to a 50-year-old beginner who wants to lose weight as it would for a 12ndlb., 20-year-old male who wants to gain muscle? No, of course not —that's why *using a one-size-fits-all program just isn't right.*

However, I won't leave you hanging. I'll give you some rough guidelines for what can be done when there is no equipment and very little time.

Isometrics are a long-forgotten form of exercise that was popular in the early and middle part of the 20th century. Isometrics are still used in gymnastics as an effective way to build strength quickly. Isometrics are a form of exercise where your muscles contract, but you don't move. Here is one example: imagine pushing into a wall.

The wall won't move, but your intention to move it will make your muscles contract.

There are two types of isometric exercise: *Overcoming isometrics* and *yielding isometrics.* Overcoming isometrics are when you try to cause motion (this would be our example of pushing into a wall). Yielding isometrics are when you try to prevent motion. These are just two examples, but you can create isometric exercises for every muscle.

You can expect some beneficial carry-over to more dynamic exercises *if you select the right exercises.* Don't expect many gains in muscle size, but you will *gain strength without gaining size.* Another upside to isometrics is that once you stop using isometrics, the strength you've built up deteriorates much slower than with dynamic exercises. In fact, you can take as much as a year off from isometrics, and still retain 80-90 percent of the strength built with them.

This is a very broad topic, and much could be written about it. Isometrics are just one option, but there are many others, like dynamic tension, more difficult body-weight exercises, special gymnastic exercises (which can be adapted to any fitness level), and many others. If you are in the situation where you habitually don't have access to equipment or for whatever reason you don't want to join a gym but still want great results, contact us, and we'll be able to set up a program for you that gets you to your goals.

It is my wish that you will gain a greater sense of how important your health is, and put it high on your priority list so that you can reap the benefits of being fit *and* healthy. As a result, you will easily *make time* for daily exercise and be aware of what foods you are putting into your body.

You know the saying, "Where there is a will, there is a way." Find your motivating factor, your "why" and hold on to it. Use the 24 hours you have been given each day wisely. You can do it!

Take the First Steps to Looking
AND Feeling Better for FREE!

www.fitnesssolutionsplus.ca

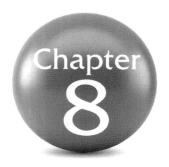

Chapter 8

Motivation: Basically, Shut Up and Get it Done!

My apologies for the rather direct approach, but sometimes you have to stop making excuses and get it done. Here's the thing: *you should not need to be motivated to exercise and eat right*. It should be part of what you do. If you say, "I used to exercise and enjoy it too, but now I just can't be bothered. Getting out of bed each day is hard enough." Your response could be an indication that you have an imbalance in your neurological or chemical make-up that is preventing you from naturally gravitating to healthy activity. See, it's not your fault! Couch potatoes are a good example of this.

Are you not as eager to exercise as you used to be and you feel as if you are just going through the motions? If you lose interest in activities you once enjoyed, and you're apathetic to most things, then it's an indication of a neurochemical imbalance.

Biochemistry in balance means you crave good and healthy food and activity. Brain and biochemistry, physiological reasons for lack of motivation, need to be addressed. The first step is to correct these imbalances. The topic of motivation is a broad topic, about which I could write an entire book (and many have been written), but let's talk about some information that is not common knowledge. After all, what good is knowing the seven things you should do (or avoid) as discussed in this book, if you don't have the motivation to actually *do* it?

Underlying Physiology

Motivation isn't limited to psychological thought processes. *There is a definite and distinct physiological component to motivation.* Your brain has certain neurotransmitters, which are chemicals in the brain, specifically designed to control motivation. One of those neurotransmitters is *epinephrine*, which is the one that gets you excited. Another one of those neurotransmitters is *dopamine*, which gives you feedback about pleasure. When you're doing something that feels pleasurable (stop thinking dirty!), dopamine is released.

Many other chemicals influence motivation, for instance low testosterone (in both women and men) and DHEA could lead to loss of motivation. Low thyroid can have the same effect on you, and there are many others.

How Do You Know When Low Motivation is Due to Physiological Imbalances?

Simply ask yourself: have I lost my motivation for exercise primarily or for other things that I normally enjoy too? If the answer is that you have diminished motivation with regards to exercise *only*, then chances are this decrease in motivation is psychological. If you're also losing interest in other activities, chances are there is some biochemical imbalance in your body. Correcting these imbalances with the help of a qualified medical professional will help restore motivation.

Once imbalances have been dealt with, you can then address the issue of normal, healthy motivation. As discussed in the previous chapter, you need to have a strong enough reason to do what you need to do.

Igor Klibanov

Have a Strong "Why?"

Let us talk a little bit more about the concept of having a compelling "why". Ask yourself these valid questions: '*Why* is exercise important to me? What is the end goal of exercise? What happens if I don't achieve that end goal? How will I feel? How will my life be different six months from now if I don't achieve that goal? How will my life be six months from now if I *do* achieve that goal? *Why* am I doing what I am doing? *Why* am I running 10K or *why* on earth am I climbing the CN tower one step at a time?'

Author Victoria Lorient-Fabish, suggested that one of the biggest mental blocks to weight loss is the lack of self-value: self-value is a feeling that you're worth self-caring. She said that people do not see the downside to their excess weight but instead see it as some sort of benefit where they have a sense of protection and safety. She suggested some strategies to help to remove those mental blocks:

- *Visualization is an effective tool.*

- *Goal setting. This is how you get self-esteem. Create bite-sized goals and then feel a sense of self-value as you accomplish the goals.*

- *Recognize the hurt child. Avoid eating to satisfy the inner hurt child. Use self-love and visualization to help and if you need it, seek therapy to heal the hurt.*

Victoria is the author of, *Find Your Self-Culture: Moving from Depression* and *Anxiety to Monumental Self-Acceptance*. She added this time management tip:

"People need to establish boundaries in their life. Having good boundaries and learning to say no helps a person build confidence and this feeling will assist a person in building self-esteem."

Bruce Krahn suggested that your goals need to evoke a feeling of excitement to keep you going. He said, "You have to be heavily emotionally invested. If you don't have that emotional investment, get mentors who've achieved what you'd like to achieve. Hang out with them, and it rubs off on you."

What Motivates You?

Actually answer this question on paper. Write it out. You know, the way people used to do before computers existed. Consider the way you think about exercise and fitness. Dr. Lise Janelle, D.C is a transformational coach and founder of the Centre for Heart Living. She said that one of the biggest mental roadblocks to body transformation is that if the subconscious mind has associated more pain than pleasure to something we want consciously, the subconscious mind will sabotage us. Dr. Janelle said, "Our thoughts biochemically impact our body."

Igor Klibanov

The most common motivators in the over 35-year-old crowd are, "I want to be a good example to my children." The other one is, "I see my parents' poor health and I don't want to go the same way." Those below 35 years old often just want to look good on the beach.

Have you thought about how you were taught to view exercise when you were a child? What attitude did you inherit from your parents? In an article for HUFFPOST Healthy Living, Dr. Lise Janelle wrote, "Up to 90 percent of what we do is actually subconsciously driven by beliefs we gathered along the way, especially in our childhood." Take a moment to think about how you view yourself, your body and your self-worth.

Your "Why" is strong enough if it evokes an emotional response, or a gut response within you to compel you to take action. Then it is a good reason to keep you going. A simple reminder, a picture or some other visual cue will remind you of your reason for working on your health and fitness.

Usually negative emotions are stronger motivators than pleasant emotions. By this I mean that although doing a 10-km race is a nice accomplishment, in my experience in the fitness industry, for many clients, the thought of losing their health - which is a negative thought - is a stronger motivator to get to the gym.

These kinds of motivators have to be felt physically and if you can combine the two motivators, even better. For example, people who have survived heart disease or a heart attack have felt the painful consequences of not taking care of themselves and do not need much motivation to stay fit and healthy post-recovery. They have an emotional as well as a physical reason to stay on track. You want your reason for exercise to evoke emotion.

Excerpt from the book called, *Switch: How to Change Things When Change Is Hard, by* Chip and Dan Heath:

"For individuals' behaviour to change, you've got to influence not only their environment but their hearts and minds. The problem is this; Often the heart and mind disagree. Fervently."

Chip and Dan maintain that when there is conflict between the two systems of the brain, which are the emotional side and the intellectual side, the emotional side will always win. Our rational side has to outsmart our emotional side in order to come out on top.

You want your reason for exercise to evoke emotion.

A good illustration they use is from Jonathan Haidt's book, *The Happiness Hypothesis,* where Haidt says that our emotional side of the brain can be likened to an elephant and the rational side likened to the rider perched on top of the elephant. Typically, the rider is in charge until the elephant decides to go against the direction and wishes of the driver and goes its own way. The driver has no choice but to go along with what the elephant is doing whether they like it or not.

Chip and Dan Heath point out that situations like this include overeating, skipping exercise, sleeping in, or saying something you regret and there are a whole lot more. The best thing is to get the elephant and rider to move together. This way, change will come about more easily. The authors, Chip and Dan Heath state that you must address two things: the emotional side as well as the intellectual side. If there is a conflict between the emotional side and the intellectual side, the emotional side will always win.

Intellectually, you may *know* that ice cream (or insert your junk food/drink of choice) is not necessarily conducive to your health, but if there are emotions attached to said food, they will often override your intellect. Sure, you may be able to use willpower for a few weeks to suppress those emotions, but eventually, the emotions will overcome your puny willpower.

Make sure that your emotions are in line with your intellect. If it's important to you intellectually, do whatever it takes to evoke a corresponding emotion. It doesn't have to be a positive emotion; it could be an emotion of disgust, anger, or sadness. As long as it is a strong emotion, it will get the job done.

For many, what triggers a response in their behaviour is seeing a picture of themselves when they were not expecting to be photographed, and thinking, "Is that really what I look like? I don't like that!" For some, their doctor has told them that if they want to see their children graduate, they'd better lose weight. For others, it may be that they have a physique that they really aspire to and wish to keep. Whatever your motivation is, just make sure there is strong emotion attached to it.

You can reprogram your mind. Here's how: go back to how they did it in the old days where you had to write out lines if your teacher wanted to encourage you to change behaviour. Write, "I will go to gym because..." Fill in your *own* reason and write this mission statement ten 10 times every day and eventually *it will sink in.*

If there is a conflict between the emotional side and the intellectual side, the emotional side will always win.

Igor Klibanov

When you get to the gym though, be sure to actually *do some exercise*. Don't just take a photo and post it on your favourite social media site. Actually get in there and work up a sweat, do a workout!

Take Measurements

Measure whatever is relevant to your goal. If your goal is aesthetic in nature, measure things like body fat and circumferences. What is the mirror telling you? Are your pants fitting better? If your goal is performance-based, measure whatever is relevant to your performance. Perhaps you were able to run a 10K in two minutes less than your last race? Or you were able to go up five flights of stairs whereas before you could only do four? Progress is still progress.

It doesn't matter whether your measurements are moving in the right direction or wrong direction; you need to continue to measure regardless of how you feel about them. If your measurements are moving in the right direction (that is, you're losing body fat and/or gaining muscle), that should make you happy. You're getting closer to your goal. Happiness is a good motivator. If your measurements are moving in the wrong direction, don't just throw up your hands and say, "What the heck, I'll have cake!" Rather, get angry. That's good too because anger is a strong motivator, and it will add to your motivation in a different way.

Have a Troubleshooting Plan

When measurements aren't going in the right direction, rather than getting angry, some get discouraged, and lose their motivation, thinking, "Maybe it just isn't worth it." If you have a troubleshooting plan on the other hand, throwing in the towel can be avoided.

Have three different plans for these three potential situations:

Your measurements may be:

1. *Moving in the right direction, so you're making progress.*

2. *Moving in the wrong direction so you're regressing.*

3. *Stagnant, so you are neither progressing nor regressing.*

If you are progressing, keep doing what you're doing. If you are either regressing or stagnating, have a contingency plan *before* you take your measurements. Don't wait until you take your measurements to start setting up a plan because if you do that, you likely aren't thinking logically. You will respond to your emotions which may not be the best thing to do. You need a clear head to formulate *a plan of action*, and when you're either angry or upset your plans don't tend to be sound.

Be realistic about how much recovery time you need between workouts. Dr. Ken Kinakin, said, "There's a level of recovery needed post-exercise. *Be patient.* Most people overestimate what they can do in a month, but underestimate what they can do in six months." Your consistency and good habits WILL PAY OFF! Hang in there.

Registered Holistic Nutritionist Lori Kennedy gives the following tips to stay motivated:

- *Set realistic daily, weekly, monthly goals.*

- *Just take it one day at a time.*

- *Have a strong motivator: picture, card, words and language.*

- *Recognize that it's a journey, not a quick fix.*

- *Have a level of self-acceptance that roadblocks will come.*

Blackmail Yourself

Yes, your eyes are not deceiving you. This is a useful strategy; blackmail can be an extremely effective motivator. One way to blackmail yourself is to have a negative consequence for failing to reach your goal. Tell everyone about your goal and chosen consequence. In the book called, *The Blackmail Diet*, by John Bear, you will read about one man who blackmailed himself in this way: if he did not loose 70 lbs. in one year, he would donate a large sum of money to a Neo-Nazi organization. This is obviously something *he did not want to do*, so he lost those pounds instead.

Your blackmail doesn't have to be quite as extreme, but the key to a successful blackmail is twofold:

1. *Come up with a negative consequence. Find some way to make sure that consequence does become a reality if you don't reach your goal. The man in the example above put his money in escrow. It's very important to make this a consequence you don't want to happen. If it's a negative consequence, but you don't really care, or if it won't have a negative impact, you will not be motivated to follow through.*

2. *Tell everyone you know about your goal and the self-imposed consequence.*

Set Up a Support System

Set up a group of people around you who will be there to support and encourage you. This stifles those inevitable toxic people who would otherwise sabotage you (who are often those closest to you). They will tell you, "Honey, you look great the way you are, so have another piece of cake." On the other hand, if you request their assistance in attaining your goal, they will think twice before tempting you. Suddenly they are on your side and on your team.

If you let your goals be known, and you fall off the track three months down the line, someone will inevitably ask you how you are progressing and it is embarrassing to admit that you fell off the wagon. The thought of having to admit defeat is a strong deterrent to giving up. Join support groups online or in your community, these groups can be invaluable when you feel discouraged or need someone with whom to celebrate a victory.

Post your goals and progress to your choice of social media sites and then *everyone* will know if you are cheating and you will have a support team. You will find encouragement and support where you least expect it.

Go ahead and sign up for that exercise class you have been curious about! You can only win by trying it out. If you have been deliberating about whether you need a personal trainer or not, now is the time to take that leap of faith and invest in your health. You know where to find us.

Once you have identified strategies that will work for you, *put them into action.* This is that part where you just get it done. Correct any physiological imbalances if need be and do not be afraid to seek help. From time to time we need to reach out and ask for help. We live in a time when stress is having adverse effects on our bodies and minds. Implement strategies so that you will be able to reach your goals and feel the satisfaction of a healthy and fit body so that you can enjoy the life you have been given. Invest time and effort into your health and fitness because you are truly worth it.

Special Opportunity for Readers of

"STOP EXERCISING!
The Way You Are Doing iT NOW."

THE MOST INCREDIBLE FREE GIFT EVER

($90 Worth of Pure Body-Changing, Performance-Enhancing Information)

Igor Klibanov is offering an incredible opportunity for you to see WHY Fitness Solutions Plus is known as "THE COMPANY" where busy professionals seeking EFFECTIVE and Dramatic Improvements go. Igor wants to give you $319 worth of pure Body-Changing, Performance-Enhancing information including a personalized Dream Body MAP Session and Biosignature Assessment. You'll receive a complete map of your body.

Dream Body MAP Session

- How any person can gain the individual blueprint to look better, feel better and perform better.

- How to avoid exercise and nutrition programs that don't work.

- The hidden reasons you can't lose weight.

- The BIGGEST MISTAKE most people make in their exercise and nutrition.

Biosignature Assessment: The ESSENTIALS towards Losing Weight Without Counting Calories and Using Iron Willpower.

- How to optimize your body fat and lean muscle mass.
- Key elements that determine your body fat.
- How to lose body fat the right way for you.
- Which food and supplements you should use to help you lose weight.

These FREE Gifts are redeemed at
our facility in
Markham, Ontario, Canada
(five minutes north of Toronto).

To redeem them, scan the QR code
below or visit:

www.FitnessSolutionsPlus.ca/dream-body-map-session/

Igor Klibanov

Eight Things You Should Know Before Hiring a Personal Trainer

1. Can the personal trainer intelligently combine exercise with nutrition and supplementation?

Most trainers are only trained in the exercise side of things. They may learn about Canada's food guide (or your local country's nutrition recommendations) and they will not learn about supplementation. If they do have some knowledge of nutrition, it usually comes from fitness and bodybuilding magazines. Those aren't good sources of education. So make sure they have some formal training in both nutrition and supplementation.

This factor is very important because you get much better results when you intelligently combine all three: training, nutrition and supplementation.

2. Make sure the trainer performs an initial assessment.

If you just come to a trainer, tell her/him you want to get in shape and she says Great, let's go", they're missing out on a lot. Make sure that, at a minimum, they ask you very precisely what it means to you to get into shape (to some people, it's to lose 10 lbs., to others it's to bench press 200 lbs and yet for others, it's to run a marathon), what your exercise history has been, what injuries you have had, what is your medical history, and what is your time availability.

Bonus points if they do a more thorough assessment that involves you going through some exercises to see how you move and what imbalances are present in your body.

As an example, in our company (Fitness Solutions Plus), we look at:

- *Your goals*

- *Your exercise history*

- *Your medical history*

- *Your time availability*

- *Your nutritional habits*

- *Your current medications*

- *Your current supplements*

- *Your hormonal profile*

- *Your muscle balance*

- *Your range of motion*

In certain cases, we may even perform some laboratory testing for toxicity, nutrient deficiencies, and hormones.

3. Ask what professional development courses they've taken.

Although I don't put much stock in certifications (or even degrees for that matter), I do put a lot of stock in a hunger for knowledge, and you want a trainer who is really on top of things.

In the past, I've interviewed trainers who had master's degrees in kinesiology, and the highest certifications in this industry. Yet, when it came to their practical knowledge and results with clients, it was sadly disappointing.

At the same time, I've interviewed people who didn't have any degrees, but their practical knowledge was astounding.

There's a difference between having 20 years of experience and one year of experience 20 times. That difference is professional development.

4. Make sure that they have an actual, written program for you (although this may be less necessary in a small group). They shouldn't just make up exercises as they go along.

After your initial assessment, the trainer should walk in with a program that they designed **just for you**, based on the results of your assessment.

This shows that they have thought ahead of time about what's right for you, and they're not just making up exercises as they go along.

It's the unfortunate truth that in many cases, personal training is nothing more than glorified babysitting.

When your trainer has put in the thought into what is right for you, and takes the time to explain to you why that program is **right for you**, then it becomes a professional service.

5. Make sure they do regular assessments (every two to four weeks) to measure progress, and adjust your program based on the measurements.

If you're not assessing, you are guessing.

It's important to measure, measure, measure. But it's important to measure what's relevant to your goals. For example, in our company, we rarely have you do pushups or sit-ups for as many repetitions as you can. Why? Because chances are you walked in with a different goal. You might have come in wanting to lose body fat or gain muscle. How many sit-ups you can do has very little relevance to those goals.

So measure, but measure what matters.

6. Make sure they write down what you did on any given workout.

Tracking your progress is very important. Chances are that you are not your personal trainer's only client. Do you think s/he has a chance of remembering which exercises you did two months earlier, with what weight, for how many repetitions, and how long you rested in between? Not a chance.

That's why writing down what you do every single workout is tremendously important.

Plus, your own training log is a goldmine of information. When you start analyzing different training programs compared to your measurements, and seeing the effects on your body, you learn very precisely what works <u>for you</u> and what doesn't.

7.   Make sure they know how to help your specific goals.

A lot of trainers use a one-size-fits-all approach. In other words, if a trainer absolutely loves bodybuilding, MMA, yoga, pilates, or distance running, they will use those approaches for every client, regardless of whether the client's goal is bodybuilding, fat loss, getting rid of lower back pain, or reversing osteoporosis. You want a trainer who knows how to work with all types of clients.

8.   Make sure they have a referral network.

Sometimes a client comes in with issues that are outside a trainer's scope of practice. So make sure that trainer has at least a naturopathic doctor and a chiropractor/osteopath/physio they can recommend to you.

Igor Klibanov

Also make sure that the trainer did the research on whom they are referring you to. In other words, very often, they'll position chiropractors in the same facility as the gym itself, and if your trainer is referring you to that practitioner, it's usually just for convenience and not because that particular practitioner is anyone special.

Make sure the trainer you're working with has thoroughly researched the person to whom they're referring you, and they're referring based on clinical excellence and not for any other reason.

Take the First Steps to Looking AND Feeling Better for FREE!

www.fitnesssolutionsplus.ca

OTHER BOOKS FROM BLACK CARD BOOKS

Let's Chat Series
Bringing Order to Chaos
Feminine Solutions For The
12 Most Common Stressors
In Life
Mehjabeen Abidi

ISBN: 978-1-927411-21-6

The Fit Bitch Diet and
Fitness Rules
Dare to Change
R.J. Tabuchi

ISBN: 978-1-927411-26-1

SOLD
The Secrets to Selling A
House Fast, For Top
Dollar, With Less
Hassles
Mehran Bagheri

ISBN: 978-1-927411-25-4

FREEPUBLICITYNOW.COM
Simple Steps For Super
Exposure
Cathy & Rick Nesbitt

ISBN: 978-1-927411-17-9

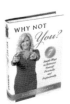
Why Not YOU?
7 Simple Ways to
Reinvent Yourself
Personally and
Professionally
Nicole Normand

ISBN: 978-1-927411-16-2

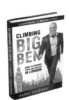
RELATIONSHIP ROI
How Associations,
Charities, and
Entrepreneurs Hit
Financial Targets
Nikki Pett

ISBN: 978-1-927411-12-4

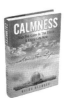
Calmness
Find the Calm in the Storm
and Enjoy Life Now
Helga DeSousa

ISBN: 978-1-927411-53-7

Climbing Big Ben
A Guidebook to Making it
Big!
Harry Sardinas

ISBN: 978-1-927411-33-9

OTHER BOOKS FROM BLACK CARD BOOKS

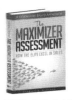

THE MAXIMIZER ASSESSMENT
How the Elite Excel in Sales
Derrick J. Navarro

ISBN: 978-1-927411-24-7

STOP EXERCISING! The Way You Are Doing It Now
7 Dangerous Facts That Will Cause You to Stay Fat or Hurt Yourself
Igor Klibanov

ISBN: 978-1-927411-52-0

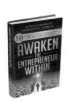

Awaken the Entrepreneur Within
10 New Ways To Think Entrepreneurially in Any Size Business
Anwar Jumabhoy & Srikrishna Vadrevu

ISBN: 978-1-927411-59-9

Investment Crash
Wie Sie finanziell erfolgreich werden in unsicheren Zeiten
Andreas Hoerman

ISBN: 978-1-927411-28-5

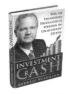

The BIG PAY OFF
Pay Off Your Mortgage Years Early Without Making More Money Or Changing Your Lifestyle
Itay Avni

ISBN: 978-1-927411-23-0

The Power Of Pets
7 Effective Tools For Healing From Pet Loss
Marybeth Haines

ISBN: 978-1-927411-07-0

The Honest CEO
The New System for Strategic Planning From Initiated to Implemented!
Johan Johannesson

ISBN: 978-1-927411-22-3

DIVORCE 2.0
The Secrets to a Friendlier Divorce
What Lawyers Don't Want You To Know!
Maureen Tabuchi LL.B

ISBN: 978-1-927411-14-8